SAVED
BY THE
BLUES

36 Stories of Transformation through Blues Music and Dancing

By

Rebecca Pillsbury

COPYRIGHT

SAVED BY THE BLUES
36 Stories of Transformation through Blues Music and Dancing

Copyright ©2016 by Rebecca Pillsbury

Cover Design by Antonio García Martín
Cover Photo by Evrim Icoz

Published by Duende Press

ISBN: 978-0-9915254-3-0

TABLE OF CONTENTS

I

SHARING THE BLUES

II

BODY

VI

SINGING THE BLUES

DEDICATION

For Sol

I remember the night we met,
at a blues dance house party in Buenos Aires.
There weren't many of us there,
but I'm glad because it gave us more time to talk.
I was so happy to meet another vegetarian.
Your passion for the earth and for animals
stayed with me.
But not as much as your spirit...
Your contagious enthusiasm for life...
Your optimism that the condition of the world
would get better.
I wanted to get to know you better.
I left Buenos Aires knowing that
I wanted to keep you in my life.
We did stay in each other's lives
for the next seven years,
though only through email and social media
and our thoughts.
We promised to visit each other...someday.
I never did make it down there again.
It still hurts that when you came here to Portland,
I was overseas.
I still can't believe that only a couple of months later—
the week we were to hold our interview for this book—
your spirit would leave your body.
You were so young.

You seemed healthy.
I hope you were happy.
The condition of the world hadn't seemed to have
gotten much better after all.
But I know you never lost hope.
You were searching for your own utopia.
You thought it might be New Zealand.
Or maybe Hawaii, or Tahiti.
I shared your love of green spaces.
We said maybe we'd meet up on an island someday.
We had a lot to catch up on.
I told you I'd written a memoir about my life
since we met in Argentina.
You were reading it the week of our scheduled chat.
We had a lot more in common
than we'd ever realized, you said.
I couldn't wait to hear more.
I was so glad we'd be reconnecting—
even if only through Skype.
The night we were to chat,
you asked if we could reschedule.
You'd recently been mugged—twice—
and understandably, you were feeling quite anxious.
I asked if you wanted to talk about what had happened,
but all you wanted was to take a bath and go to bed.
That's what I would have wanted to do too.
We said goodnight.
"I promise we'll Skype this week," you said.
But I had an uncomfortable sensation
that we might not.

I brushed it aside.

A few days went by. I didn't hear anything from you.

But I got a call from a mutual friend.

What he shared broke my heart.

You are one of the most joyful, loving spirits

I've ever met.

No one who meets you forgets you.

You're still alive, I know.

Not only in the hearts and memories of all who loved

you but in the air.

In the earth.

In the sun.

Thank you for sharing your gorgeous light—in bodily

form and in spirit.

I know we'll meet again…someday.

I can't wait to dance with you again—

like the night we met, when neither of us had any idea

how to lead.

We laughed and did side-by-side Charleston instead.

Remember that?

I'll never forget it.

INTRODUCTION

Melancholy. Despondency. Depressed spirits.

These are the words you'll find if you look up *blues* in the dictionary. Whether pertaining to someone having the blues or someone playing the blues, the believed common denominator is sadness. But go beyond knee-jerk response to the word and think about the times you've actually listened to the blues. Did the music make you feel sad? Or did it release some of the tension inside of you? Playing the blues, listening to the blues, or dancing to the blues is used as a means to *overcome* sadness.

The blues isn't about self-pity; it's about empowerment. It celebrates ownership of anguish, rather than avoidance. It recognizes that to feel pain is to be human and that only by fully experiencing the intensity of this human emotion can the pain be transcended. Sadness—and the coming together in community as a result of that sadness—is not seen as tragedy but as beauty.

This is part of what makes the blues therapeutic—it distracts us from all of our desires, including the desire for our suffering to end. To cease desiring relief is to find relief. But don't take it from me; read the thirty-six stories in this book from people all over the world—people who have found healing through playing, singing, or dancing to the blues.

This book is divided into six sections, with each section dedicated to a central theme. The reader will notice some crossover within many stories that means that story could just as easily belong in a different section—one aspect of the human experience affects another, which affects another, and so on.

As much as our individual facets are interrelated, there is a variance of personal experience and culture. One contributor may have a very different perspective on the same topic than another—including the appropriate name for the dance style this book is about, or the characteristics that define it. I've chosen to let each contributor use the definition most relevant to him or her, be it *traditional blues*, *alternative blues*, *fusion*, or simply *blues*.

This book is not to serve as an academic study of the dance itself or dance therapy but rather to offer various personal experiences throughout each individual's journey of transformation.

But before we talk about the powerful end results blues music and dancing has had on so many individual lives, let me share a bit about how the music and accompanying dance forms began.

The Roots

Traditional blues music originated on the plantations and in the cotton fields and gin houses of the Mississippi Delta in the late nineteenth century. It evolved from the spirituals, work songs, and field hollers of African Americans enduring slavery and sharecropping. However, we could trace its roots back even further—to two distinct strains of music from West Africa.

One strain, from the Senegal-Gambia region, was more rhythmically complex and incorporated the Arabic propensity for long, tortured melodies. The other strain was that of the Congo-Angola region, which was more vocally rich and refined, involving call-and-response singing, or field hollers. Field hollers would begin when a lead worker chanted an opening line and the chorus of workers answered, falling into a regular pattern to match the task at hand. These chants made the work day go faster and brought people together in community.

The vocal expression of distress was joined by stringed instrumentation, introduced by traveling musicians of West Africa known as griots—a hereditary caste responsible for maintaining the oral history of their tribes and villages through stories, poems, songs, and dance. In both West African regions, music played a communal and often dance-driven role, serving as the focal point at religious rituals, during planting and harvesting, while dwellings were built, and for celebrations.

Upon being brought to America during slavery, the musical traditions of Africa mixed with Western classical and folk traditions, including instruments such as piano and guitar, and becoming what is known today as blues music. Much of this original blues music, unfortunately, followed these early musicians to their graves. However, their influence and legacy can be heard in the recordings of some of the first well-known blues musicians of the 1920s and '30s, including Son House, Blind Lemon Jefferson, Charley Patton, and Robert Johnson. Listen to a recording of Blind Willie Johnson's "Dark was the Night, Cold was the Ground" and not only will you be brought back to the early blues era but you will be powerless to its ache.

The adoption (by force) of the Christian faith by newly arrived slaves led to a deep influence of the gospels on blues music. Many of the legendary blues musicians have some connection to the Christian church. Son House was himself a fallen preacher—a teenage pastor who became a prison inmate ten years later—and Robert Johnson is famous for his encounter with the devil at "the crossroads," where he supposedly sold his soul in exchange for his ability to play the blues.

These musicians typically performed solo with just an acoustic guitar, although they would occasionally team up with fellow bluesmen, or blueswomen—the 1920s and '30s also gave rise to female vocalists, including Ma Rainey, Bessie Smith, and Mamie Smith.

In the post-slavery era, racism, extreme poverty, and devastating natural disasters led to the massive diaspora of African Americans from the South to northern cities such as Chicago, St. Louis, and Detroit. During the early to mid-twentieth century, the blues continued to grow and evolve, reflecting the changing circumstances. While the guitar remained the central instrument, it became electrified by blues musicians such as John Lee Hooker, Muddy Waters, and Howlin' Wolf and was accompanied by instruments such as the drum kit, piano, harmonica, and a variety of horns.

In the 1950s, B. B. King introduced a sophisticated style of guitar soloing based on vocal-like string bending and left-hand vibrato, which has influenced countless electric blues guitarists and rock guitarists alike. King and his style of electric blues contributed to opening blues music to a wider audience, especially white listeners, narrowing the gap between the African American community and mainstream American culture. The performers themselves also grew to include white guitarists and vocalists, like Stevie Ray Vaughan, Eric Clapton, and Bonnie Raitt in the 1970s and '80s.

The urban blues scene began to enthrall listeners who were black and white, young and old, rich and poor, and every possibility in between. What made the music of one group's struggles and strife so universally appealing?

The blues sings of the universal themes of love and loss, work that is often repetitive and unsatisfying, and trying to find strength in misfortune. It reaches out to all, naturally drawing people together during times of hardship. The narratives build mutual solidarity, creating a space that is communal and intimate. Its listeners are provided safe opportunities to be vulnerable—to share their most authentic selves. The blues says, "This is all of *me*, and I see all of *you*. Let's take our individual stories—our own blues—and create something of beauty together."

The Church

Not everyone saw the emotional cleansing, self-expression, and sense of community that blues music and dancing evoked as positive, however. The Christian church was less concerned with overcoming adversity and improving the quality of everyday life than it was with salvation of the soul after death. Trials and tribulations were, after all, meant to be endured in accordance with the will of God. The blues musician's ability to generate joy and merriment through methods other than the teachings of the church was considered sacrilege.

The music was referred to as "devil's music," for church elders and ministers believed that its expression led to behavioral temptation in conflict with the scriptures. To them, to play blues music was to call the devil to come forth and reign upon earth. Internal and external conflicts tormented members of the community who participated in the Saturday night ritual of music and dance and the Sunday morning ritual of worship. Their Saturday night practice was one of purification, just as was their Sunday morning practice. Both experiences purged the heart and mind of sadness and strife. But the dance hall remained, to church elders and ministers, a house of sin and folly and eternal damnation of the soul.

Of course, some churches were not void of their own style of good-time music. Spirituals often ignited eruptions of clapping and shouting, rocking and rolling, foot shuffling and ecstatic revelation. However, the dance style that the spirituals evoked was different than the style evoked in the dance halls, or juke joints. The dancing in the juke joints had an added element of sensuality—not an expression in congruence with the Christian church.

It wasn't in agreement to incorporate religious elements into blues music, either, but it happened nonetheless—sometimes through lyrical arrangements but other times because the deep power of the blues lament naturally invokes an experience of the divine. The ability to call forth the divinity within us—to generate our own source of healing—gave rise to fear in the church. If we didn't rely on the church for community building and healing, church leaders perceived a loss of control—not only of parishioners' individual lives but in the whole structure of society.

The Transformation

So, what is unique to the blues that allows for such a powerful emotional response that the depths of one's soul can be accessed and healed? In a word: tension. Emotionally expressive music tends to create a degree of tension, such that finally experiencing its release is cathartic.

One of the ways tension is created in the blues is through pitch bending. The vocalist or musician slides his or her voice or instrument up or down pitches of a key, such that the notes "bend" to create a sense of uncertainty and anticipation. The exquisite timing of a "blue" note seems to be capable of activating an inner space in the listener where emotions such as loneliness, sadness, separation, and fear are stored. When the target note is eventually reached, the tension is released, and often a state of euphoria is experienced.

We aren't necessarily conscious of this delicate interplay, but blues lovers nonetheless experience it. For the keen ear, that bent note on an electric guitar has the potential to take your breath away. Around that note, the wailing cry of a harmonica can make you want to cry out yourself—in pain or pleasure—and the solid rhythm of the drum beat can bring you back home as it reverberates in your soul and reminds you of your roots.

The intricate musical techniques used in the blues are, therefore, capable of turning negative emotions into excitement, and by doing so transform trauma into ecstasy. The blues performs a cleansing of the soul. The song builds up tension, seeks and finds release, only to build and seek release again—just like the human experience of life itself.

Nowhere is the intensity of musical potential more profoundly felt than while listening to a live performance. Unlike a classical musical performance, which is celebrated for its exact rendering of the score, a blues performance is revered for being different every time. Just like life, the song is ephemeral, ever changing, and nontransportable, and therein lies its beauty. Let's celebrate *that*—this experience we're having *now*, because it's not going to last.

The great musicians of the world are able to evoke such powerful reactions in their audience not simply because they're able to effectively express their own pain and sorrow—it's because their listeners are suffering too. With all its "blue notes" and overtones of sadness, blues lyrics feature the most harrowing hardships, anxieties, and misfortunes. If listeners pay them heed, they are sure to find commonality in experience. In a sense, their attention is being drawn to their own fears and insufficiencies.

Despite the dark themes that blues music encompasses, its nature and function remains a form of entertainment—its purpose is to make people feel good. Even when the vocalization and instrumentation express the most miserable moaning and groaning, and the lyrics depict pain and suffering, blues music often serves as the conduit for the high point of a festive occasion—offering a dimension of down-to-earth sensuality that makes people want to get up and move.

The Dance

I've spoken of dance halls as venues for blues music and dance revelry, but the shacks in which the blues began its transformation from a form of self-expression into a form of entertainment were more often called juke houses, or juke joints. The word "juke" originated in the West African Congo and means "evil, disorderly, wicked"—in many traditional African societies, close couple dancing was considered immoral. Since absorbing into English, the word has come to refer to sinful pleasure. Juke houses often doubled as brothels and were places to drink, gamble, wreak havoc—and dance the blues. It is no wonder, therefore, that churchgoers associated the blues with sin.

The dancing itself was no less free of "inappropriate" behavior, by church standards. All that slow dragging, belly rubbing, hip grinding, and flirtatious strutting became synonymous with the blues, and synonymous with sin. The more lowdown and dirty the music, the more sensual—and sexual—the dance moves.

Apart from being more sexual, the dance was known for its unique combination of spontaneity and improvisation, while still maintaining a sense of control. It shook off the more stylized versions of ballroom dance and became more rhythmic and fluid. Although often practiced with a partner, the dance was more an expression of the individual's personality and soul. The music allowed the soul to access not just its primordial sensuality but the joyousness, exhilaration, and delight in human existence. The dance was an opportunity to symbolize and stylize one's own perceptions and feelings in response to that music.

A dance-beat-driven personality cannot *not* dance when a blues song is played. Once phonograph records were created and radio networks began to broadcast dance music, there were more blues-oriented bands on the road than ever before. Even when blues music was performed as a vaudeville act, the audience was foot tapping and hand clapping and doing whatever other dance-inspired movement the facility's space allowed.

W. C. Handy, who wrote some of the first published blues songs, described what happened when he played "St. Louis Blues" for the first time in 1914: "When 'St. Louis Blues' was written, the tango was in vogue. I tricked the dancers by arranging a tango introduction, breaking abruptly into a lowdown blues. My eyes swept the floor anxiously; then suddenly I saw lightning strike. The dancers seemed electrified. Something within them came suddenly to life. An instinct that wanted so much to live, to fling its arms to spread joy, took them by the heels" (Handy, 305).

For black or white or rich or poor, the blues has the universal ability to recreate the emotional landscape of life and to help relieve the weight of its daily burdens. Whether a person was dancing at juke joints alone or with a partner or taking in a musical performance of the blues at a variety show, the emotionally and rhythmically charged lyrics and melodies of the blues offered a release of tension that would carry that person through the week...until it was time for the next fix.

The contemporary blues dance scene looks decidedly different than the scenes in the juke joints and vaudeville venues of the twentieth century. The blues dance scene—and even that term—as we know it today evolved out of the swing dance revival of the 1990s and early 2000s. All across the United States, and also in Europe, multiday swing dance events—Lindy Exchanges—catered to the new, primarily white, aficionados of the black vernacular dances of the 1920s–1940s. The organizers began hosting late-night "blues rooms"; after the exhausting physical demands of a full day of Lindy Hop dancing, dancers would migrate over to the slower, smoother style of dance that blues music inspired.

Another style of partner dance has recently evolved from the contemporary blues dance scene, referred to as "alternative blues," or "fusion." Although related to blues in its improvisation, the music is not necessarily that of traditional blues, and the dance movements themselves may draw from outside the blues aesthetic to incorporate elements of tango, Lindy Hop, contact improv, and even ballet. This dance style has grown in part due to Blues Recess dance events being held around the world in both rural and urban locations. These community-driven gatherings lean more toward experimental movements and alternative lifestyles than does the traditional blues dance community, although the magic in dance connection is much the same.

Blues dancing, therefore, is difficult to define; just as the music itself is constantly evolving and being influenced by what is popular of the day, the dance movements are adapting to influences from different cultures, new adaptations of blues-rooted music, and each dancer's own personality. Blues dances as a genre, however, tend to share an aesthetic that includes: a grounded body posture where the weight is held on the balls of the feet, the knees are bent, the hips are back, and the chest is forward; an asymmetric and multirhythmic movement among body parts; improvisation on an individual level and between dance partners that may incorporate call and response; and dancing in the space between the beats—creating a sense of tension in the body while remaining loose and relaxed.

And one key trait defines these dances—that is intimacy. Danced most often in close embrace, the dance is raw, vulnerable, and exposed. Like the music itself, the intention is not to hide or avoid who you are and what you're going through but to face yourself and your partner fully—and by doing so transcend time, space, and fear. No matter if what you're dancing is a variation of traditional blues or alternative blues, there is healing that takes place.

Exposure to the healing power of the blues is no longer limited to the United States and Europe. Modern-day blues dance scenes are developing around the world, as a result of individual dancers and instructors traveling between local and international communities and hosting blues dance workshops and "blues exchanges." These events serve the purpose of not only familiarizing communities with dance styles evolving in other parts of the world but offering a sort of cultural and social exchange.

Local dancers host visiting dancers, and non-dance events are often held throughout the day that provide an insider's view of the local culture and an opportunity to connect in a meaningful way with people from all socioeconomic, generational, and racial backgrounds. Thus, healing doesn't just take place on the dance floor—as human connection is made across cultures, our similarities are recognized, our differences are celebrated, and a new level of acceptance is achieved.

The Book

I've outlined a brief history of blues music and dancing to offer a context in which readers can better understand what is to come. But this book is not actually about what blues music or dancing is or where it came from; it's about how it feels—which is something different for everyone. Despite the variance of experience, however, there are commonalities to be found. The blues experience is, again, within the larger context of a shared human experience.

The idea for this book was born at the Rose City Blues dance event in Portland, Oregon, in November of 2013. I had just written my first book—*Finding Ecstasy*—which is a memoir that details my own journey of healing through blues dancing. There was a moment during the headlining performance of the night by the legendary Curtis Salgado when something in the music—perhaps now I could distinguish it as a particular display of vocal tension—caused an emotional and physical, and I'd say spiritual, reaction in the audience that led to newly partnered dancers separating, rushing toward the front of the stage, and breaking down in solo movement, reminiscent of a down-home church gathering during revival time.

I was in the midst of the revelry myself, having my own transcendental moment—but something caused me to turn around and take in the experience of the room. Hundreds of dancers faced me, eyes closed, arms raised, clearly feeling something very powerful. I knew what I was feeling. But what were they feeling? What were their stories? I wondered. Through the writing of my memoir, I knew how therapeutic it could be to reflect on one's own journey, to shed the veil of anonymity and publicly announce, "This is who I am, *fully.*" By doing so, so much inspiration can be found in one's challenges and triumphs.

I suddenly had a driving impulse to offer others that experience. I began writing this book, therefore, as a platform to explore and honor people's personal stories and to inspire readers through their journeys. However, amid the interview process, a dear friend—who was going to be a contributor to this book, and to whom this book is dedicated—experienced a fatal heart aneurism after an assault. While processing my own grief of her loss and the circumstances around it, I realized this book was really about something else—or rather, something more.

Tragically, the world is becoming increasingly one of fear, isolation, competition, and repression—emotions that lead to such human behavior as theft, assault, rape, and even murder. How can we attempt to heal such a world? Global healing has to begin within each one of us—and here's why I believe we can begin by dancing.

Throughout the more than forty interviews I conducted for this book, a theme recurred: the importance of human connection, the experience of oneness with other human beings. Within each dance, there is an exchange of the purest form of love. When we truly *see* the person in front of us, we can't possibly hurt him or her. When I go dancing, I look around the room, and I see dance partners spanning all faiths and cultural, racial, and economic backgrounds. They are smiling at each other, holding each other, *seeing* each other. In a dance, you're simply two human beings exchanging something pure, fulfilling the need for human connection—a sense of belonging, of contribution.

My hope is that this book will inspire more people to dance—to step outside their comfort zones, to shed not just their anonymity but their own beliefs about how human differences set us apart. If dancing can provide an opportunity to be fully seen and *still* loved…can you imagine the effects on humanity?

I'm not saying that dancing is going to solve all the world's problems…but wouldn't it be a great place to start? So, what do you say? Let's transmute tragedy into beauty. That is the essence of the blues, after all.

Let's dance.

I
SHARING THE BLUES

Everyone has a personal reason for wanting to share his or her love of blues dancing with others. For some, it's to encourage a healthier, more physically active lifestyle. For others, it's to develop deeper, more meaningful relationships. It can also be used as a means to travel the world, establish a new career, or ensure that a family tradition lives on. The contributors to this section were inspired to take on leadership roles in the blues dance community for these reasons and more.

Elsa Zanzibar, for example, decided to organize a blues scene in Paris, France, because she wanted to bring the magic of the experiences she'd encountered dancing in other countries to her hometown. Like other dance organizers I've known, she actually moved to a different home in order to comfortably accommodate dance guests. She shared her reasoning. "Hosting is a better way to know people than meeting them in a workshop; you get to know them deeper. Also, it forces you to change the rhythm of your normal life; you learn to take time to enjoy the benefit of their presence."

Vicci Moore, one of Europe's only full-time dance instructors, along with her partner, Adamo Ciarollo, agrees. "As blues dancers, we have a bed-and-breakfast in any city in the world; the people blues dancing attracts are generous people. You have to be a giver to be a blues dancer."

Sometimes their dedication to sharing the blues with others can consume their professional and social lives. But what keeps them giving is that they get so much back. Vicci concluded, "The students inspire me so much. I can't imagine doing anything else."

She can remember, however, what it was like to be doing something else—living in London without feeling part of a community. When she first discovered the blues dance world, she wondered, "How long has this world existed…and why didn't I know about it until now?" She does not want that same circumstance to befall others looking for connection, self-expression, or any other element of the human experience they may feel is missing from their lives.

My deepest gratitude goes out to all those mentioned in this book—and the many more dance teachers and organizers out there who sometimes work so hard to make dance available to others that they don't have much opportunity to dance themselves. As demonstrated in the following pages, there's no telling how far their efforts reach.

Keeping the Dance Alive

Damon Stone, Minneapolis, Minnesota, USA

Damon came to my attention through another contributor who knew I wanted to talk with someone who taught traditional blues dancing—the family of historical steps danced to blues music before the 1960s. As someone who is passionate about not letting the roots of the dance die, Damon is eager for an opportunity to teach not just the dance but its history.

Damon's introduction to blues and jazz music began in a unique way—while watching cartoons. "When I was about six years old, my grandparents were babysitting me. I was watching a TV show that repeated the chorus from an Ella Fitzgerald song. When it was over, I was skipping and dancing around the house singing that song. My grandmother asked me if I wanted to learn how they used to dance to that style of music. That became my introduction to solo blues and solo jazz movement. For the next few years, playtime became putting on music and dancing."

As a preteen and teen, he danced with his relatives at family gatherings. Then various family members invited him to join them at blues clubs in their home city of Chicago. There, he was excited to see people not related to him doing the same dances. These African American dancers were people like himself that had learned these steps from their families or communities. Since "blues dancing" is a contemporary term, they probably would have referred to the dancing they were doing to slow music as just "slow dancing."

After moving to San Francisco in his twenties, Damon learned about the area's significant underground swing dance community. "San Francisco was one of the hotbeds in the underground swing scene—you had to know somebody who knew when and where a dance was going on." This growing community consisted of people who had begun to study early jazz steps, like the Lindy Hop.

The faster jazz steps Damon grew up learning were the same he saw others using in San Francisco; however, it was the way he moved to slower blues songs by artists such as Count Basie, Duke Ellington, and Cab Calloway that caught other people's attentions.

"I started dancing the way I'd learned from my family. People liked it and wanted to learn how to do it. There was only one other guy in the community at the time who was well versed at dancing to that kind of music—another black man who also grew up learning the dance from his parents, who learned it from their parents.

"Other people's interest spurred me to start asking questions rather than just copy what my family members were doing. 'What's the name of this? Where does it come from?' I remember the distinct point I transitioned from wanting to learn the dances from a social perspective to wanting to learn them from an academic perspective: when I was reading *Jazz Dance* by Marshall and Jean Stearns. The back of the book has a list of all these different dances and what they're connected to, and it has some choreographic mapping of how blues dances were done. One of my great-aunts asked me what I was reading, so I explained it to her. I'd say a name of a dance, and she'd say, 'Oh, I remember that one,' and her and my uncle would get up and start showing me the different dances. They became my dance mentors; that was probably around 1996 or 1997."

There was no recognized blues dance community that he was aware of at that time. "A blues dance scene didn't develop until probably 1998, when you'd see DJs and bands purposely playing slower songs."

He related that, at that point, "there was not a lot of distinction between what I was doing on the floor to slow music and what people who were really good swing or ballroom dancers were doing, except for quality. For most of them it was something very new, whereas the people I learned from had been doing it for decades."

He explained the reason the commonalities outnumbered the differences: "The concept of musicality—of what makes this music distinct from another and leads us to move in a fashion that compliments that particular musical element—is what distinguishes one dance from another. Once you understand the music, dancing is just moving your body with another person."

Damon credits the introduction of a blues dance community in the United States to a town distinct in many ways from American cities: Herräng, Sweden. The town of just over four hundred inhabitants is home to the world's largest annual dance camp, which focuses on African American jazz dances. Although the camp centers on Lindy Hop dance instruction, in the late 1980s, it began hosting weekly blues nights.

Damon believes that the camp organizers weren't referring in their naming of these nights to the dancing or the music necessarily, but rather they wanted the nights to encompass the same feel as a juke joint—a music club popular with African Americans in the southern United States in the 1910s to 1960s. Damon attests that the music itself wasn't strictly blues but a "mix of slow jazz, soul, funk, and rhythm and blues with traditional and hyphenated styles of blues music that was more emotionally evocative." From there, Americans began bringing this idea to the United States.

Blues rooms began popping up at Lindy Hop exchanges around the country, leading to a growth of interest in the dance as its own style. Damon recalled the first exclusively blues dance event held in the States, in St. Louis in 2003. It was a one-day event for people in the region, but it expanded over the years into a multiday event with instructors and students from across North America—including Damon. The success of this event led to additional blues dance events springing up around the country.

Initially, Damon was hesitant to consider himself a teacher. Friends had asked him to teach them how he danced as early as the mid-'90s, but he was uncomfortable accepting money. Eventually he agreed to show them what he knew—borrowing phrasing and concepts he'd picked up from his family and from swing instructors he'd had, including dance legends such as Frankie Manning, Norma Miller, and Chester Whitmore—only if they paid him not in money but in sushi. "I like to say I taught for tuna rolls," he stated with pride.

Soon eager new students began approaching him. Key swing instructors in the local scene took note, and when gigs came up that required them to travel on weekends, they asked Damon to take over their classes. They insisted on paying him with money. Over fifteen years later, he's still teaching and traveling the world as a popular dance instructor.

Rather than "blues," Damon calls what he teaches "jooking," to refer to the dances he'd learned that came out of Memphis juke joints and back-alley blues clubs. By doing so, he attempts to avoid confusion as to the style of dance he teaches—the definition of blues dancing varies depending on who you speak to.

Damon posited the following: "Blues is not a dance; blues is short for 'blues idiom dance,' and there are a very large number of African American vernacular dances done to this music—slow drag, savoy walk, Texas shuffle—every one of which has its own basic individual step. But if I don't recognize them as individual dances and I see someone shifting back and forth between the dances, I might not recognize there are multiple dances being done.

"Therefore, for a good decade, there was a lot of debate around this idea that 'blues dancing' is whatever you want it to be, that it had no rules. But there is not a single street dance that has ever developed on this planet that doesn't have rules. By their very nature, dances have borders, in the same way that languages have borders. You can create something new within those borders—colloquial expressions, new words or pronunciations, but if they don't adhere to the functional and artistic aesthetic, it ends up being a different language."

Damon feels rather passionate about the topic; he had to defend his stance quite a lot among other burgeoning instructors in the early years of the blues dance movement. That debate prompted him to explore what academics were finding in regards to historical African American dances. "More and more people started making academic research available, and it became easier to find certain video clips that showed this kind of dancing being done to that kind of music, and it became harder and harder to say there were no rules. If there are no rules, how do the leader and follower communicate? There would be no reason one should take lessons."

The foundation of what Damon and other traditional blues dance instructors teach has since become the norm on the national scene. However, he still is concerned about the roots of the dance aesthetic dying out. "Not that there won't be something being done that has some sort of association to traditional blues dancing, but it won't look like how it began."

Damon paused to reflect back on how his own dance journey began, and why it's so important to him to keep this style alive. "It started out with just having fun. It was a way to spend time with my grandparents and get energy out. When I became a teen, it was about getting a chance to dance with all the pretty women. As I got older, it became a matter of loving the movement itself. Now, as some of the people who taught me are passing on, my goal is to try to keep the dances that I'd learned alive. It's a way to give thanks for what they've passed onto me, a way of honoring their memory."

Damon could even say he owes his existence to his grandparents and other relatives in more ways than just blood. "I was raised with dancing. I wouldn't even say it's part of my identity; it's more fundamental than that. I don't go around saying, 'I'm a breather,' or, 'I'm an eater.' I could no more live without dance than I could live without food or water or oxygen or sleep; it's fundamental to my existence. Every aspect of my life has been touched by dance. I am who I am because of it."

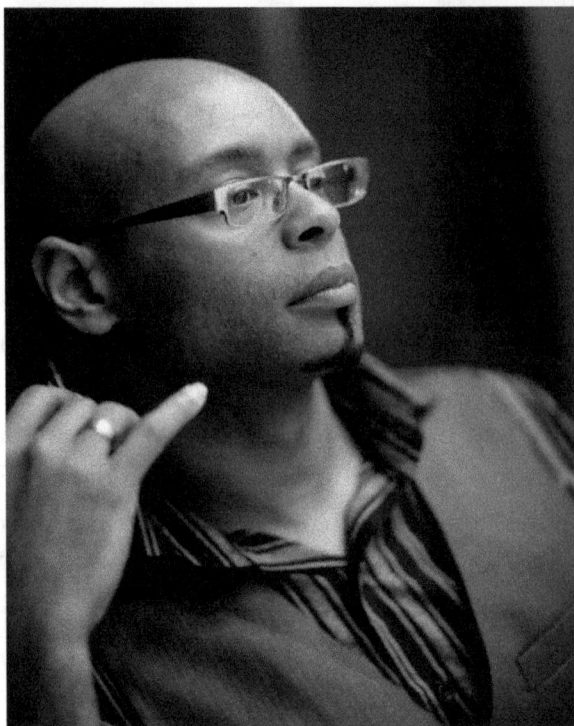

Photo by Bobby Bonsey

An Ambassador for Movement

Brenda Russell, Portland, Oregon, USA

Brenda has been an ambassador for blues in the Portland community since what has come to be known as contemporary blues dancing began—or what she refers to as the blues dance subculture. She will tell you that, like Damon from the previous essay, she and members of her family were "blues dancing" before that term even existed—they simply called it "dancing." What is more important to Brenda than what you call it, however, is the fact that it makes you move.

Brenda is a movement educator certified in the Franklin method, which promotes ideal functioning of the body and mind using motion and imagery. She does this through teaching various styles of dance—from Lindy Hop to salsa to blues—and by incorporating her knowledge of martial arts, yoga, anatomy, and the healing arts into her lessons. Her classes are no longer confined to the Portland area—there is a high demand for her lessons across the United States and Europe, and she spends half the year traveling to accommodate that demand.

Movement itself has always been really important to Brenda. "When I was three years old, I told my parents, 'When I'm an adult, I'm not going to have bad knees and a bad back and neck. I don't think adults should be in pain.' My parents didn't know where I got these crazy ideas."

She grew up in a home where movement was encouraged. She recalled having heard very different messages at some of her friends' homes, stern demands like "Sit still" or "Stop fiddling around." Brenda, on the other hand was allowed to climb on furniture and jump on the bed. "My mom called me Monkey Do because I was always swinging on things in the house. I was a wild kid physically in that way, so those messages I heard from other parents really stood out to me."

Brenda was a natural dancer and a natural teacher. "I was labeled a teacher at about nine years old, within multiple communities. When I joined the dance community as an adult, within six months, people were asking me to teach. I felt that you should be dancing at least ten years before you teach, but everyone was telling me, 'You get it faster than everyone else, and you know how to break it down—just help us.'"

Brenda wasn't just getting asked to teach dance steps in general; also like Damon, she was getting asked to teach how *she* dances. It all started with swing dancing. "Within the swing dance community, there were these house parties that we were having really consistently. At the end of the night when the DJ started playing slow music, I'd start to dance, and people were like, 'How do you do that? What is that you're doing? We want to know how that works.'"

So Brenda began teaching blues dancing—but she called it "groove." She explained, "We were doing so much more than traditional blues dancing. It evolved to be something very different, but I do understand that the roots are the same—the part that we are healing and rebirthing ourselves through movement. There is an emotional intensity to the music, whether you're listening to electronic music or Howlin' Wolf or Robert Johnson; there's a sense that we are unburdening ourselves through the music, and that's the same regardless of how we're dancing to it, or what we are dancing to."

Brenda noted that the music and the dance generalized long before the contemporary blues dance scene did so. "There are over fifty countries in Africa, and every village has its own dance. So when African slaves from all over the continent were brought to America and began sharing their cultural dances, the dances got mixed up. However, there are specific steps that people have documented with a similarity among them, only stylized differently.

"I feel like it's the same way for blues dancing, different types of syncopated steps, ball-chain steps, certain movements of the spine, undulations, isolations, and certain ways of swinging the body. I think that for me, what I've seen and what I've experienced, the steps that are done in traditional blues are very similar to what I've seen in traditional African dance steps but adapted to the music of the day. The styling changes a little bit each time that it's done, since it's expressed as it's felt in that moment, but the base is the same."

Brenda concluded her description of blues dancing: "What we think of as blues dancing is what people in the past just called dancing. It's how we dance when the music is slower." And how we dance is based upon what we feel—which is driven by the music. She offered a theory on why music has the power to evoke an emotional response that moves people: "Blues music has this intensity within it because of the timing of the rhythm and the stretch. There's always that tension and release, that mournfulness and angst. I feel like those emotions are inherently within blues music."

Like fashions or other trends, there is a natural ebb and flow to what kind of music generates popularity or interest at any given time. With the rediscovery of swing and big band music in the 1990s came a new surge of people interested in swing and Lindy Hop dancing—music that was popular in the '30s and '40s. This trend also led to renewed interest in traditional blues music.

"The Lindy Hop community was building, and people were always doing some kind of slow late-night dancing. It was a time when people were starting to look back and learn more about these traditional dances. Social dance was getting lost in our culture, and there were people all over the world researching it. In any movement, there's always the grandparent, and then the next generation and the next generation, so I feel like by the time we got to the early 2000s, there was more of a critical mass, and the contemporary blues scene really kicked off with blues house parties."

Some dancers join the community for the simple love of the music or for the freedom of expression in the dance. For others, the community satisfies their desire for human contact. It is not uncommon to find a group of dancers snuggled in a corner. Although romantic and sexual relationships of various natures do develop from such circumstances, it is by no means the rule. Often, people are simply craving intimacy—not to be confused with sex—a topic Brenda feels strongly about.

"I'm shocked by how many people say that intimacy and sex are the same thing. It's sad, really sad. People often don't understand that you can have intimacy with a nonsexual partner." The perception of a lack of distinction between the two likely originated in the church and is why blues music came to be called the devil's music.

"There is this religious programming that sex is of the devil, dancing leads to sex, and sex is bad. So the idea that blues music is related to the devil, of course, that makes perfect sense. As soon as you start to move with undulations and isolations, that's considered sensual movement. In order to feel your body, to love yourself and heal yourself with movement and with touch, that would be seen as leading you toward sex— it's opening you up to be sexual."

Along with being an ambassador for movement—particularly within the blues dance world— comes Brenda's offshoot role as an agent of change in how sex and relationships are perceived in our culture. She is saddened by the belief that we still live within a sexually repressed culture. If sex is a consensual decision, Brenda questions why it can still be perceived as "bad."

"The idea that we can play this music and move our bodies and make choices around sex that are not unhealthy for us just wasn't part of the cultural thinking at the time when blues was considered of the devil. Now, with the more modern way of thinking about sex, people are definitely more open and logical and enlightened. These ideas are becoming more widespread, so hopefully it will shift."

In part due to the practice of open or alternative relationships that some members of the blues scene participate in—more often on the US West Coast—Brenda feels that shift is imminent. "I really see members of the blues dance subculture as relationship pioneers. There are some negative side effects to the extreme lifestyle that some of the people in the subculture live, but there are also some really groundbreaking and beautiful things happening."

Fulfillment of sexual expression or intimacy aside, it cannot be denied that there are many powerful healing factors taking place on the dance floor and within the dance community. For those looking for a scientific explanation of how dancing affects physical or emotional health, there are several resources available (some of which are listed in the back of this book). This book is about personal experience, and in that respect, Brenda can testify as a witness to the remarkable transformations she's seen take place.

"I saw pretty early on as a dance teacher that when I would ask someone to do a certain movement, it would bring up a lot of emotion for them. There were parts of their body they could move easily, and parts of their body they couldn't move at all. And if I kept encouraging them to move the parts of their body that were restricted or stuck, then a lot of times tears, anger, and hesitation would come up. They would start asking questions to distract, you could see the ego jump in there to try to protect.

"I can see the healing power of dancing in my private lessons and my group classes. I've taught people moving through huge transitions in their lives and those moving through small, momentary transitions in their lives." She went on to offer an explanation for those shifts. "Moving the body moves energy—it releases energy. People in cultures all over the world have been using movement to heal the body since forever. In addition to teaching dance, I'm a medical chi gung practitioner, which uses movement as a healing practice. Those familiar with reiki or somatic psychology will have heard the term 'armoring.' There are various famous psychologists, like Wilhelm Reich, who suggest we hold trauma or tension in our bodies in different places, and when we try to move, it can be really intense emotionally.

"Even in yoga there's a sense that certain misalignments in the body are related to certain emotional things, or what Louise Hay calls in her book *Heal Your Body* 'metaphysical causations.' It's very interesting what can happen in just one hour of doing what is basically a type of somatic therapy—you go and try to move your body in a way you haven't tried to move it in a long time, and all of a sudden there's a flood of emotions that have been unaddressed."

Brenda's experience has led her to develop a strategy to deal with this situation. "You have to start really small, really slow." One of the first things she does with a new class is watch how students move their bodies to a beat without being told what to do.

"I teach a Katherine Dunham class—she was a modern dancer who has a method based on African movements—where we use drums and do movement for the entirety of the class, and I watch and see how the students move their bodies. The drums are going crazy, and some of them are just jumping and flailing, with a lot of movement happening and a lot of energy releasing. But for other people, movement is barely perceivable; you watch them and it just looks like they're standing there, lifting their arm or kicking their leg or slightly wiggling their body. They'll be sweating and sore the next day and will feel really invigorated with their endorphins going, but for them that's as much as they can handle at that time. So it takes some time; it takes a safe space to break through some of those things."

Brenda is careful, however, not to use only free-form dancing in her blues classes. "I think that doing both prescriptive steps and doing free-form movement is healing in different ways. When you do a prescriptive step, you find out where you're stuck, and when you do free-form, you let your body go where it wants to go—which means that it might find an area that it's not ready to deal with, or it might go somewhere that it *is* ready to open up. In all movement modalities that I've studied, we do a combination of prescriptive steps and free-form."

Especially for people who have lived more sedentary lives, it is true that dancing can sometimes lead to injury, but typically dancing is not the cause itself. "I've had students who get an injury within the first few months of dancing. I know now through the studying I've done that those problems started before they started dancing, and dancing just accelerated them to flare up. The injury is forcing them to look at what was going on in the body all along.

"That's where dance is healing and therapeutic for people—they are learning a lot about themselves. I think often that's what leads people to the dance floor—they're trying to heal themselves. We have a large percentage of people who just got out of relationships, who had some kind of recent trauma or loss in their lives, and they're looking for some type of connection, some sort of healing."

Brenda has her own personal dance and movement practice as well, which is often conducted to live music. "I go out dancing almost every night. I try to dance to live music at least one hour per day. I want to support live music and dance being together. I actually feel like the healing power goes up pretty significantly when there's live music involved with the dancing, so I'm really focusing on that aspect.

"My dance classes have live music most of the time now, and I want to continue working less and less with recorded music. In general, I'm just going through life being an ambassador for movement, and that means I'm willing to stretch or wiggle or dance in public places where other people aren't doing that. I try to find that balance, where I'm not being rude or inappropriate but instead trying to shift cultural ideas and expectations."

Brenda can't ensure such a shift alone, although she's doing everything she can within her capacity to spread the word. "I'm writing several books on dance right now. One of those books is about having a home movement practice—how to create that practice for yourself, without putting that responsibility on someone else. We may need to have a teacher or mentor for a period of time before we're willing to take ownership of our own practice, and that's okay, but eventually moving to that space where we take responsibility for our own health and wellness is the goal. From there, the teacher's role becomes more about feeding or instructing your personal practice."

Reflecting on Brenda's concept, I began to consider that it's the same for our dreams—we can't materialize them by sitting and waiting for them to come true. For many people I've met on the dance floor, their dream was to learn how to dance. Once they've learned how, they want to do it forever.

"Everyone was so inspired by Frankie Manning dancing in his eighties and nineties. Everybody wants to dance until they die. So how can we do that, how can we dance until we die?" Brenda's answer to that question can be witnessed in her students.

"I look around my classroom and see all these people out there moving and dancing, and that's exactly what I feel my mission in life is—to support them in a movement-based lifestyle. They're not sitting on the couch watching TV—they're out moving, and I'm so excited about that."

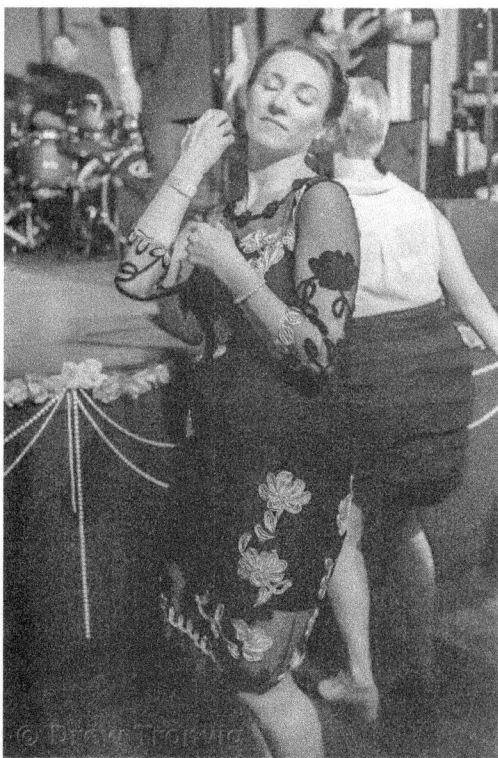

Photo by Drew Tronvig

There's No Such Thing as Someone Who Can't Dance

Dave Madison, Dance Nomad

For the avid traveling blues dancer, Dave is a man who needs no introduction. He's one of the early founders of the contemporary blues dance scene. Here, Dave shares not only about the evolution of the blues dance scene from house parties but about his own personal journey of discovering everything from a welcoming community and a new career to the love of his life—all through blues dancing.

Our discussion began with a brief history of the blues dance movement, and the role he played in its development—starting with his own infamous house parties.

"We started having house parties in San Francisco where people said, 'Let's do that dance thing we've been doing at the end of Lindy exchanges.' So the scene started off with just Lindy Hoppers—usually ones who traveled a lot and were pretty experienced dancers—who began showing up for these house parties."

It spread from there; dancers who had traveled from Portland, Seattle, and other cities began hosting parties at their homes. Large groups would carpool to the events, sometimes traveling great distances. "We started getting people from as far as Texas and New

York and then they would go back and host blues dance parties in their communities."

What started out as intimate gatherings began to grow exponentially. "Our finale in a sense was a three-day-long house party that had hundreds of people show up and many bands, so it basically became like an exchange event. At that point, a dancer from San Francisco contacted me and said, 'Why don't we have a workshop on the Friday before your party?' So he brought in these people to DJ, and he held a workshop. That led to the start of an event which turned into Friday Night Blues, which is the longest and oldest running weekly blues dance of the contemporary blues dance scene. I think that's where the formalization of the dance as its own culture started."

Dave's personal journey to dance started well before then, when a friend suggested they watch the movie *Swing Kids*. "I didn't dance until I was twenty-four years old. I'll never forget that night—there's this opening scene in the movie where they go through the doors of the Bismarck in Hamburg, Germany, and everyone's dancing, and *boom* everything clicked for me. I knew—*that* is what I'm doing with the rest of my life." What he hadn't known was that his friend was an avid swing dancer. When the movie ended, she got up and started teaching Dave how to dance.

"We danced for four or five hours that first night, just learning. Then the next night, and the next night, and the next night." He hasn't stopped since.

Before dancing, he hadn't made time for much outside of the fifty to eighty hours he worked each week as a computer engineer. "I was dumping my life into my job. After that movie night, everything in my life has been dedicated to dance since then." Including his subsequent move to San Francisco because "it was the best place in the world to do the kind of dancing I wanted to do."

Even though he still poured himself into his career upon moving to San Francisco, he made time to dance nine times per week. And not just locally: "I started traveling for dancing *a lot*, which is not great for a career outside of dance. Suddenly I was taking all my vacation time just trying to do these extended weekends." He soon realized that the high he got from dance was not the same he got from his computer work. Around the same time, the company he was working for in Silicon Valley went under. He considered it the perfect opportunity for a major shift in the way he lived and worked.

"I wanted more to my life than just some job that I did. I didn't want to be my career—I wanted to go and experience life. What I wanted to do is what I do now. I work in spurts, doing an intense amount of work, and then I have a huge amount of freedom to travel. I live in a tour bus, which is often in storage somewhere while I'm traveling around Europe. I spend about half the year in Europe, so my life from a pragmatic perspective has completely transformed. Now, I'm wandering the world, and I've seen and experienced so much."

Where he travels is dictated by where he gets a teaching job. Even if there is no established blues dance scene, Dave can help start one. He excels at teaching beginners because he remembers what it feels like to be one himself. "I've only met one person who had more trouble learning how to dance than I did. Anybody can learn how to dance—it just takes practice. I know it because I've seen it. For the last fourteen years, I've been analyzing dance pretty seriously from a teaching perspective. It can absolutely be taught to anybody. There's no such thing as someone who can't dance."

And once you start, you never know where it may lead. "Dancing has changed everything in my life. Aside from where I spend my time and money, one of the things that's changed my life fundamentally is having this extended family." The latter is one attribute that keeps Dave comfortable in and committed to his nomadic lifestyle. Wherever he goes, he feels welcomed and at home.

"I think there's a filter that happens for people who are drawn to dance. The vast majority of people who are drawn to dancing have this innocence in their hearts that they bring to the dance floor. People who go out partner dancing want excitement and connection in their lives. They're looking for something—maybe it's love, or maybe they're just looking for more essence in their life than most people I see living."

What Dave gets from dancing goes beyond career and lifestyle and relationships. It's a state of bliss. "Dancing allows you to get 'in the zone.' There's a natural physical state your brain gets into where it's able to get lost, and that's a really pleasurable place to be. There's a high you get from it—the endorphin or serotonin rush. There are some times when I feel so lost with somebody; I'm dancing with someone, and the connection is so great, and we're feeling the music so deeply—everything is just *working*. We're creating something that is beyond what our brains can process. I guess some people get to that same place through meditation, some people get there through drugs or sex or religion. Each has their benefits and drawbacks, but dancing will generally get you healthier at least." Dave paused before reconsidering with a snicker. "Although if you do it as much as I do, it can destroy your body."

I decided to wrap up the interview by asking Dave what he thought his life would be like without dancing. His reaction makes me laugh every time I recall it, although there was nothing on his face but fright as he replied, "Oh, geez. Oh my god. That's terrifying. Wow. That is like a horrifying question. Oh my god."

Finally, he laughed before continuing, "I'd probably still be working and looking for friends and for loved ones. I think it would have gotten so bad that I would have had to search for something at some point. I think some people are content to live your basic standard life, and some people need something more than—or different than—that. I didn't even fully understand how much I needed something different until I found dancing. Dancing gave me everything in the end.

"It's brought me love and heartbreak so many times. All of the big joys and pains in my life have in some way been related to dance for at least the last ten to fifteen years. I found my fiancée because of dance. Dancing gave me this interesting and fascinating life, it gave me a way I could travel the world, it gave me a career where I could get paid to teach, it gave me all this family and all these friends, and it finally gave me my loved one. I mean…there's nothing else I really need at this point."

Dave wanted to make something clear, though. "But it's not like I found my love, so I don't really need dance anymore. My fiancée is a dancer too, so we will always have dance in our lives. We'll always have each other to dance with. And I'm guessing that we'll always have blues in some way."

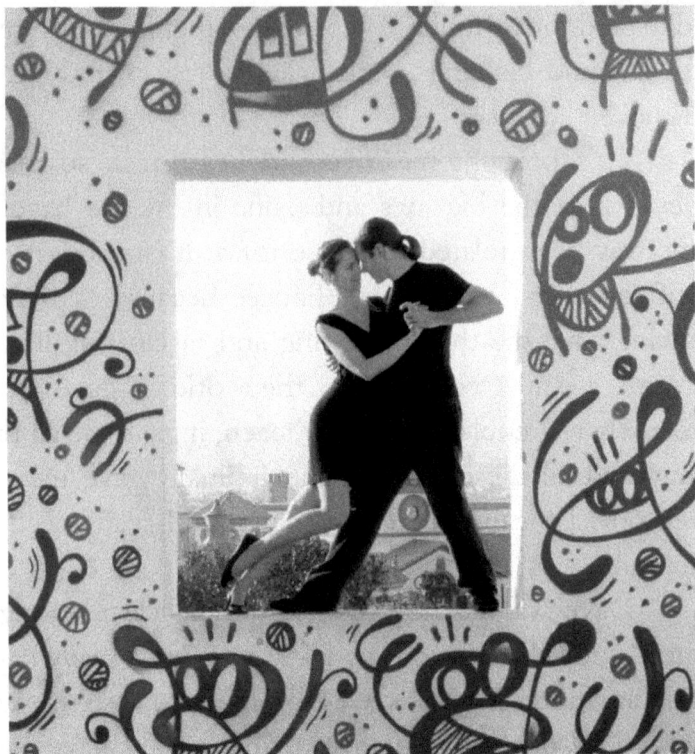

Photo by Nuria Aguade

My Alternate Life as a Dance Organizer

Nadja Gross, Zurich, Switzerland

Nadja first came to me at the European Blues Invasion to share eye-witness accounts of the transformations she'd seen in other dancers. Several months later, however, I approached her about sharing her own story—as well as offering insight into the growth of the blues dance scene in Europe. I had seen her tireless efforts organizing her own events, and I was intrigued by her motivation.

Nadja has organized the Blossom Blues dance festival in Zurich, Switzerland, since 2012—a weekend of blues dance parties and classes preceded by one week of an intensive blues dance camp. The event attracts dancers from all over Europe, as well as from the United States.

Nadja's introduction to blues dancing began in Boise, Idaho. She had just completed her master's degree, an accomplishment she celebrated by taking six months off to travel in the United States. She was staying with friends in Boise when she decided to attend a dance class.

Nadja's initial hesitation to the close embrace of the dance wore off before long. That embrace, in fact, is one of the things she has come to appreciate most about the dance. "That's what I love a lot about blues—even with people you've never met before, you dance with them in close embrace, it feels wonderful, and then afterward you say good-bye and you never see them again. For me, that's one of the most special things. You don't really get this connection in other ways—you have to get to know a person and find out about common interests to feel a connection, and on the dance floor it happens and you don't even talk."

Although regular blues dance events were already taking place in other cities in Europe—most notably, London and Berlin—the opportunities for Nadja to have those profound experiences in her home country were few and far between. "There was almost no blues in Zurich. I didn't feel like I was progressing at all, so I started traveling. That's how I got to know the international scene in Europe, which at the time was still very small. I think there were three or four weekend workshops, and if you look at it now, there's something going on almost every weekend. So I got on the blues train when it was taking off."

Nadja is one of the reasons for that acceleration. For the past four years, she has been organizing small local workshops as well as the large annual Blossom Blues event. Her strategy is to bring in high-quality instructors and to experiment with what modules inspire the most integration among community members.

This past year, she incorporated two significant—and highly effective—strategies. The first was not to divide the classes by level, an approach she'd seen employed at Blues Recess events. "Instead, the instructors gave demonstrations and then dancers chose their classes, which is a lot more social because you get to know a lot more people—not just those who are at the same level."

The other unique characteristic was to use live music for the classes. "It adds so much to the lesson when you have live music—it's incredible. The musicians love to interact with the dancers. The instructors and the musicians work together to prepare the classes, and the musicians play faster or louder, depending on where people in the room are at."

With the growing number of blues workshops taking place around Europe, it has become increasingly important for organizers to set their events apart in such ways. And they have to make more of a statement about the type of event they're hosting—be it traditional blues, or alternative blues, or a Blues Recess event, which are focused more on community building.

Despite the variety of opportunities abounding, Nadja has experienced more collaboration than competition. "There's a constant interaction among the European organizers. We talk about what we do for our events, and we give each other pointers. It's like a little group that is trying to help each other out. We sometimes even share instructors because we're bringing instructors from the United States, and it's expensive, of course, so if you can share instructors, it's good for everyone."

A more recent observation is that an increasing number of Blues Exchanges are popping up—events which do not have classes and instead incorporate time for the hosts to share highlights of their city and culture with visiting dancers. This kind of environment allows for really close relationships to form among dancers, which increases the desire to continue the traveling and dancing lifestyle.

Even though Nadja maintains a more traditional office job, the "dance nomad" lifestyle is one she has embraced. "I have friends all over Europe—really close friends, even though we live in very different parts of Europe. If someone had told me before that I would spend this much time and energy and money on dancing, I would have told them they're crazy." In fact, her friends and family sometimes think that she is—but she ascertains the dance is what keeps her from going crazy. "It's sometimes hard to explain what it means to me and why I do it. If you're not dancing yourself, you can't really understand it. I try to explain to them it's more about the community and that dancing gives me a lot of energy. Blues dancing is relaxing—it's calming in a way. I tell them I need this, that I would go crazy if I didn't have it anymore."

It's not just family and friends who have a hard time making sense of Nadja's passion for dance. "I work in energy data management, so it's a very computer-based office job. My coworkers have very different lifestyles than my own. I think some of them are jealous when I tell them next weekend I am going to Madrid or London or Barcelona, but then when I get back and they ask me if I've done certain sightseeing things and I say, 'No, I was just dancing,' then they are a bit skeptical about it again."

Thanks to her own efforts, Nadja doesn't always have to travel to blues dance anymore—or to visit with her extended dance family. They come to her. "The initial reason I started organizing is because we wanted to have blues in Zurich. But then, of course, when I get good instructors to come for a workshop, a lot of my friends come to my hometown to dance." Interestingly, however, Nadja ends up having very little time to dance herself at the events she spends all year organizing.

"The process I'm still working on at the moment is that I have to share more of the tasks. I can see that I can delegate more, let go of some of the responsibility and trust in other people to do a good job."

She has already come a long way in both her personal and professional development as a result of organizing dance events. "Every event I do, I get more confident, and I'm less nervous about it. I just know it will work, which was not always the case." No matter how stressful overseeing such an event can be, there are always moments to remind her that it's worthwhile.

"At least once or twice during an event I look around and say, 'Yes, this is why I'm doing this.' I put all this time into planning classes that I want to take, and then I don't have the time to take them—but when I walk by the class and see people really enjoying it and having fun learning together, that's always a good experience for me."

It's not just the dancers whose satisfaction offers Nadja a rewarding experience—it's the musicians' enjoyment. What's interesting is that many blues musicians aren't aware that a parallel dance scene exists. It can be hard, therefore, to find a band that is the right fit for such an event.

"We have a lot of blues bands in Zurich but not a lot that are good for dancing. So I have this one band that I contacted a while ago. They'd never played for dancers before, but they really liked the idea, so they put together a different band that just plays for us once a year, and they're *loving* it! They tell us it's the highlight of their year."

What makes the experience so memorable for musicians is that dancers are more acutely aware of musicality. Nadja described the interplay she's witnessed between musicians and dancers: "I remember the first year this band played for us. As a dancer, you know when a break is coming up, and the band was so surprised by how the dancers picked up on the break that in the middle of the song the singer said, 'Oh my gosh, this is amazing!' They'd never experienced that before. When you play for an audience who is listening so closely and clapping afterward, it's a very different kind of appreciation of their music."

Although it can be easy to observe a physical response to the music among dancers, there can be subtleties to the dance—what are sometimes referred to as "microblues"—when minimalist movements are barely visible. It is this reason that leads Nadja to believe that "blues would never be a successful competition class. You cannot see what makes blues dancing so great and have that be expressed in the competition. A good connection is not necessarily visible."

But it's incredibly apparent to those for whom it really counts: the dancers.

"I've seen some people come to a local workshop or a social dance for the first time, and they're very shy. You can see in their body language that they're holding back or even guarding themselves. Then, I've seen how this gets shaken off over time, and they're much more open and confident and outgoing."

Because she's seen the growth, Nadja does her best to encourage people who have not been dancing before to try it out. Her patience will be tested, however, if she is met with too many questions. "I had a friend the other day who agreed to come to one of the parties. She wrote to me several times asking, 'What do I have to know? What do I have to wear? Can you give me some pointers?' I was like, 'Just come! Why are you asking me all these questions?'" She laughed at her own agitation.

Her impatience can be validated by the fact that blues dancing is truly something you have to experience in order to understand. Perhaps one day her family and friends and coworkers will become curious enough about Nadja's alternate lifestyle that they'll be inspired to try dancing themselves. Until then, she will keep working with the community she has helped build to create the best events—and memories—she can.

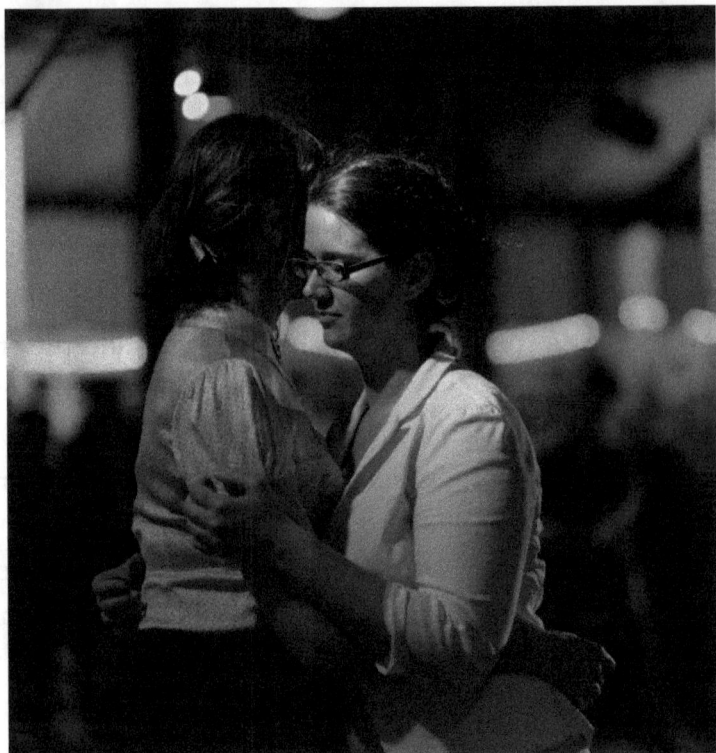

Photo by Benoit Guerin

Can't We Just Dance This Out?

Kenneth Shipp, Nashville, Tennessee, USA

My first memory of Kenneth will always be a sweet one. I'd recently relocated for just a couple of months to Nashville—a city I'd once called home. In fact, it was there that I'd first learned about blues dancing. Eight years had passed, however, since I'd last frequented the Bourbon Street Blues and Boogie bar downtown, and when I showed up there for a monthly blues dance, I recognized no one. Kenneth recognized me, however. As the president of Blues Dance Nashville—which promotes traditional blues dance classes and dances—he made it his business to welcome new dancers to the scene. He'd seen my social media RSVP to the event and wasted no time in approaching me to introduce himself.

Perhaps it was Southern hospitality or the intimacy of the scene, but I hadn't felt so welcome upon entering any new dance community before. I was introduced to all of the other dancers there that night, who made sure I felt integrated—and that I made it back safely to my car at the end of the night.

Despite Kenneth's eagerness to make me feel welcome, his natural tendency was on the quiet side. Even though I danced with him several times during my stay, it wasn't until we sat down for this interview that I learned anything about his life or the personal obstacles he'd had to overcome to dance—and to teach—blues.

Kenneth's dance journey began with swing. Nashville hosts outdoor swing dances in the summer, which a group of friends had invited him to. Soon after his discovery of the dance, however, his job in the air force required that he leave for basic training. When he came back, he found that his friends' skill levels had grown well beyond his—and he lacked the desire to try to keep up. Then he found out about blues house parties. He was intrigued. But at the first house party he attended, he uncovered a perceived conflict.

"Being a Southern Baptist Christian kid, I was like, 'Ahhh I can't do this.' There was this part of me that felt completely ostracized from my faith when dancing that style of dance." After later watching a video of a teacher exhibition, however, he discovered that the dancing at blues house parties can be vastly different than the more traditional blues style demonstrated in the video—which he loved. He was inspired to travel to see what blues dancing resembled in other communities.

The Knoxville Lindy Exchange was coming up, which he knew had a late-night blues room. He immediately recognized that the quality and awareness of traditional blues dancing there far exceeded that in his hometown of Nashville. Kenneth has since taken it upon himself to do something about that. He had to gain experience first as a dancer and then as a teacher. He knew he had to attend a workshop that was exclusively for blues. The next event he could attend was in upstate New York, in the middle of winter. He braved the cold, all in the name of blues.

Kenneth was a bit apprehensive about not knowing anyone at the event, nor knowing much at all about the dance itself. "I was really nervous arriving at the doorway to the dance. I had my nervous face on—I don't know what it looks like, but people tell me I have it—so somebody pulled me onto the floor almost immediately. When that dance finished, I got asked again, and again, and I later realized I'd been dancing two hours and I hadn't taken a break. So that did it. That solidified it for me." The community, the dance, and the music drew him in deep.

It didn't take long for him to grasp the dance itself. "Easy is not the right word to describe blues dancing, because that would cheapen it. But I think for me, I get it better than I do other dances. And the music itself, hearing how a guy is having a horrible day, or a girl is talking about how her husband left her, or whatever song it might be, I'm like, yeah, I can relate to that pain. So maybe that's what's coming out in my dancing. It just feels right. That soul stuff just clicks for me."

Like many dancers, one of the things Kenneth appreciates most about dancing is how it takes him out of his mind. "When I dance blues, I'm not thinking about what I'm going to do next or who's going to be there. At Bourbon Street Blues Bar the other night, I got to the table, I put my shoes on, and as soon as the next song started, I was dancing to the blues. Someone else had to order my beer because I wasn't thinking about that."

Kenneth doesn't require a dance partner to get up and dance, either. "I used to have to be dragged onto the dance floor, especially if it was to dance solo. Sometimes I'd dance solo by myself at home, but I was like, 'I can't do that in *public*.' But at a dance event once I saw a woman out there just rocking out by herself. I was like, 'Wow, she's in the music. She's not doing this for anybody else—she's there for her.' That really stayed with me. I'm not self-conscious about it anymore."

It can take a lot of courage to get out on a dance floor by oneself, and it can take even greater courage for a man to dance with another man. Kenneth has overcome that fear as well. It is common in the blues dance scene to break from the typical gender roles of male leads and female follows and ask a member of the same sex to dance. This practice, in addition to sometimes feeling more playful, can help improve one's own typical dance role because oneexperiences the feel of the opposite role.

Kenneth remembers what it felt like the first time he was asked to dance by another man. "I'm not going to lie—it was weird. Now I'm totally fine with it. I love to experiment with being a follow myself. I'm not good at, but I love it."

When I asked if it was his faith that had made dancing with men difficult, he replied, "My faith gotten more complicated because of dancing but not because of gender roles. There's nothing inherent in my faith that says the guy has to be the creator in the dance and the girl has to be the one following. Once I wrapped my mind around that concept, I didn't feel like my faith contradicted two men dancing together, or a woman leading a dance."

Dancing has made him look at his faith differently, but it wasn't the first time he was forced to analyze the beliefs he'd been raised with. "Basic training had already blown up my perception of my faith. I kind of had it in this nice pretty little box, and then basic training was like, 'That's not how it's going to look. This person's faith looks like this, so how are you going to interact with that?!'"

What dancing has done is expand his awareness even further. "The scene brings in so many different types of people and thought systems, so you can't be narrow-minded and dance. Well, I guess you could be, but I don't know if you're going to get the full experience that you could. If you're like, 'No, that person has to be like this, and I can only interact with that type of person,' you're not going to have a lot of fun. Even if you disagree with another person, I think you need to be flexible. You can leave it at the door—you can come out here and dance without bringing that disagreement into the picture."

In fact, that strategy is one he believes could work wonders in the military. "I think if enough people had those Zen, peace moments that I get out of blues, it might help the world to chill out. If there were blues dancing in the Middle East, we could all just blues dance together. 'Yeah, yeah, I know you guys have your different beliefs, but can we just dance for a minute and then work this out?'" His proclamation may sound lofty, but to those who have experienced the human-to-human connection that happens on the dance floor—without necessarily taking note of religious, cultural, or gender differences—the possibility feels more real.

Since Kenneth's mind has opened up, however, it has made some activities in his life harder, such as dating. "I'm a Christian guy, so I have to find someone who is Christian and who is okay with me being in the air force and with me being a dancer. And is okay with me being a *blues* dancer. That's a tall order. It's made the search parameters narrower. Dancers get it. They're like, 'Oh, they're just dancing,' whereas someone who hasn't been immersed in the scene is like, 'Ahhh! What are you doing?' I want to tell them, 'Calm down—you just have to untwist your boxes.'"

He's doing his part to spread that message to others in the local scene. "If there's any way I can help people get over issues they may have with blues—I mean, we're in the South, so if I had the issue of, 'Ewww,' when I first started, someone else is going to have that same issue—if I can help people get over that, it will be a much easier transition to building new scenes. I'd like to see the blues landscape in the South continue to change. I'd like to be able to go to different towns and find a solid blues scene there."

That goal is what led Kenneth to serve as president of Blues Dance Nashville. "I joined the leadership team because I didn't want to see blues die out again. We have way too much music in this town to not be dancing blues. That's a crime."

The role is providing him with bonus professional experience as well. "When there are thirty or forty people depending on you to have the door open, the AC on, the lights on, the sound system set up for the DJ, your coordination skills get pushed to the max. You have to learn how to delegate, learn what people's roles and skill sets are best suited for, and how to sell them on doing that."

Kenneth teaches this on a micro level too. "As a lead, I can dance and do a whole bunch of moves, but if I'm not listening to my follow, then I might as well have been solo dancing. What's the point? They have a role to play too, and I have to be receptive to that.

"If my follow wants to try something new, I'm going to give him or her the space to try that out. I tend to find out that what that person contributed is a lot better than I could have imagined. Even if they do the same thing you were thinking, letting them act builds the relationship better than you nipping it in the bud.

"I want to share these things I've learned. I don't want to tell people that dance will make you feel better, because that's almost like calling it a drug or a crutch. But I have had some bad days, and I barely remember them because the day after I was able to get a dance in somewhere. It helps—it's a way to express yourself in a different way.

"I know a lot of people say blues is not for them, but I would challenge them to start looking deeper into the songs. I'm willing to bet there's a blues song that will match something that's going on in their lives. You may not like all the songs, but there's a set of songs somewhere that's just for you, about something that you've dealt with. And if not, you can make a twelve-bar song real quick to fix that."

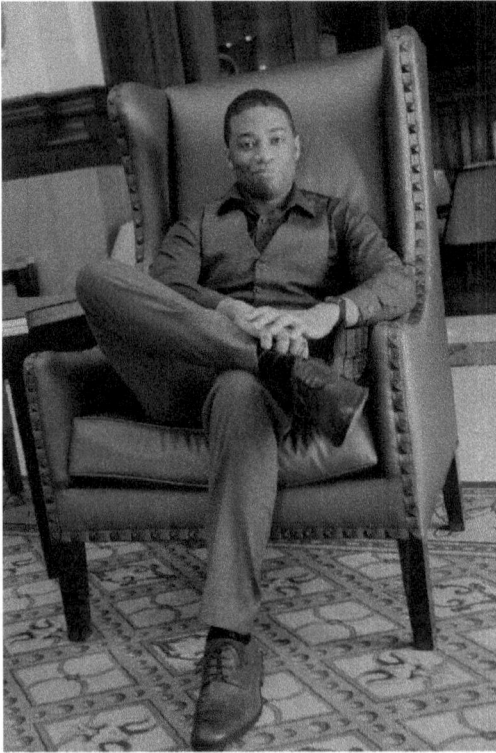

Photo by Yugandhar Beesetty

Making Every Dance Amazing

Andrew Sutton, Sacramento, California, USA

I'll never forget my first dance with Andrew. It was one of the very first blues dances in my life, in fact. I had traveled to Memphis, Tennessee, with a group of Lindy Hop dancers from Nashville, where I was living at the time. The 2007 International Blues Challenge—a highly renowned competition among the world's best blues bands—was taking place, and we planned to "blues bomb" (take over the dance floor) various venues that weren't a part of the event. We arrived late at night to our first destination. There was a small dance floor, but it was big enough for our group of ten and an additional ten or so Lindy Hop and blues dancers who had traveled for the occasion.

Andrew was one of them. I didn't know who he was at the time of our dance, but I was left awestruck. "Who was that guy?!" I remember asking a friend of mine. Of course I could have asked him directly, but the intensity of the dance had stolen my voice, and I was too intimidated to approach him again. I found out his name and that he was from Sacramento and then promptly forgot about him until years later, when he showed up at a dance in my new hometown of Portland.

The memory of that first dance came flooding back. "Did you know you're partly responsible for the devotion I've felt to blues dancing over the past six years?" I asked him. He vaguely recalled that night in

Memphis, and even less having met me. Single dances don't usually stand out for him because he aims to live a life of memorable dances.

Andrew is an internationally known dance instructor with a World Championship title to his name. His teaching method revolves around the concept that we can "make every dance amazing," no matter the level of experience. Every aspect is negotiable—that is, we can choose what we offer each partner and how we react to what each offers us. This is a key concept around the dance style Andrew refers to as "fusion." Others have called it "alternative blues"; still others just call it "partner dancing." It began in the contemporary scene, however, as simply "blues."

Andrew is not averse to the community calling the dance "blues"—but believes it would be more valuable to define it further. "Otherwise, to me, it's historically inaccurate. Rather than saying, 'This isn't blues or that's blues,' it's better to refer to the form as 'American Blues,' 'European blues,' et cetera—whatever for you defines the way you're doing it." The name given the dance form and subculture can be a triggering topic for many of its members. There is a key distinction, however, that has led Andrew to refer to the dance as "fusion."

Let's start with his experience and introduction to the dance itself. "For me, it all started with a dance event Dave Madison was holding at his house in San Francisco. A group of Lindy Hoppers came together to improve their understanding of leading and following and musicality as well. In order to break down the dance, it helped to have slower music, and blues music tended to be slower, so somehow it got started being called blues. To me, there was no reference to an old style of dance—it wasn't something we were trying to re-create based off something someone else had done, other than maybe Lindy Hop.

"But before long, a couple of people came out and said, 'That's not blues dancing; let us show you what blues dancing is,' so they started showing the steps from the early 1900s that were originally called 'slow drag' or 'juking.' So then there became an offshoot of people who were trying to recreate this dance that was done a long time ago. And I love that—I love re-creating dances—but it wasn't what I was personally going for."

It took Andrew a while to figure out what he "was going for," but eventually he realized it was a dance style that "fused" his own movements with his partner's movements, with the music. He understood that any dance could do that, but the difference for him was that fusion dancing makes those interactions the priority.

"When you make musicality and connection the priority, rather than the steps or aesthetic, it changes how you teach, how you organize events, how you dance, everything. So that's what fusion is to me, and what the contemporary blues movement was all about when it started happening fifteen years or so ago."

Andrew's introduction to dance in general began well before that, when a cute girl from college invited him to a dance class. He didn't much like it at first, however. "I felt so awkward slow dancing, or out there on my own. I didn't know what to do. It wasn't until later that I saw the deeper code; you could communicate with a partner without having to say anything, and that was extremely fascinating to me."

His interest in girls became secondary to his drive to learn more about all facets of this new language. "Once I discovered the concept of musicality—the idea of making this communication fit with the music—it blew my mind."

Andrew sought out every class and every teacher he could. However, he noticed that his teachers seemed to have conflicting points of view about what dance connection and musicality were and how to teach them. This caused him to seek out some answers: is there a universal truth about how to teach these concepts to someone taking a dance class?

Years later, after having both taken and taught dance classes in over two hundred cities and thirty-five countries, he is still in search for an answer to that question. "I have this idea that there is a universal truth, but it could be like science, where we never know the fundamental truth. That's what my search with dance has been about—are the things we think of as fundamental, *really* fundamental, or is there something deeper that will help us understand the dance more and help us connect with more people and connect to more styles of music?"

Andrew is so highly motivated to discover that truth because he wants to be the best teacher he can be. Becoming a dance teacher wasn't part of his original life plan; his college courses were devoted to the sciences. "My degree was in engineering, but most of what I was learning was not of interest to me. I didn't go to any classes—I went to my midterms and my finals, and I studied as much as I had to in order to pass my exams, but most of my time was spent on dance." His choice to continue with his engineering degree despite his lack of interest in the material was because he didn't think it was possible to make a living doing what he really wanted, being a full-time dance teacher.

Several gradual steps led him to realize that dream was, in fact, possible. The first was a series of dance classes he took, which had the students serve as teachers to one another. "For example, someone who had taken a Charleston lesson taught me what they had learned, and I, in turn, taught it to someone else moments after I learned it. That was the structure for me for the next year of learning; every week we were just sharing with other students what we had learned."

The next step came as a stroke of luck—a popular local dance instructor was moving away and needed someone to take over his classes. Andrew had just spent a summer filled with intensive dance study; he had traveled to major workshops and even performed in a local dance troupe. He was beginning to gain recognition in the Santa Barbara area and was asked to serve as the teacher's replacement. "That was the stage where I began teaching on a semiprofessional level. Still, I wasn't teaching my own concepts—I was teaching his material—but how I taught it was my choice."

His big break came soon after, while performing in his local dance troupe. "One of the most popular Lindy Hop troupes in the world was scouting for new dancers to join their troupe. I had seen this troupe perform the year before, and I was awestruck. I talked to some of the instructors, who told me how they traveled the world to teach dance, and I thought that was *so* cool. But it was a pipe dream; there was no way in my mind I thought I would ever do that." The leaders of the troupe were so impressed when they saw Andrew perform, however, that they invited him to join their troupe.

Andrew was elated. "It was a whirlwind of an amazing dream come true. I began traveling around the United States to teach dance, so that gave me the realization that it's possible to do it professionally. My understanding had been that dancers were struggling artists, living very poor lives. But I saw members of the troupe living comfortably; they weren't even the best dancers in the world—they were just really smart at the business side. So I realized I had to learn a little bit about business if I want to do this professionally."

If he were to be able to make a living as a professional dance teacher, he needed to have some titles to his name. The world championships for Lindy

Hop were being held in Herräng, Sweden, at the conclusion of a monthlong dance camp. "To me, if you went to Herräng, you became a superstar. So I decided to attend all four weeks of classes and then compete at the world championships.

"Going there, I was a whole different person. I was timid in my own scene in California; whereas when I went to Herräng, I was no-holds-barred. I was in every jam circle; I was dancing every single night, going all out." He also taught a couple of classes. The camp schedule carved out space for anyone—no matter that person's dance experience—to teach a class on a topic not taught in regular classes. Andrew decided to practice honing his skills teaching fusion.

The event set him up perfectly to make a career as a professional dance teacher. His dance skill level improved dramatically, he gained experience teaching, and he earned that title he'd so eagerly sought. Andrew placed second in the world championship competition. He was correct that a title would open up new doors for him. "Within ten minutes of the competition being over, a couple who ran one of the biggest dance camps in Europe hired me for their camp in France the following year."

Andrew returned to Europe a year later for what was going to be two months of travel. During that time, he began teaching classes in various communities, only to be asked to teach additional gigs elsewhere. "I ended up staying in Europe for over four months, teaching nearly twelve gigs, and that's when I realized I can do that full-time. I had a group of contacts then, and I started setting up my own gigs. It snowballed to the point where I literally traveled somewhere different in the world every week, for twelve years straight. It was pretty crazy, pretty fun. I loved it."

Andrew spoke in the past tense because he's set the travel lifestyle behind—at least for now. He's issued himself a new challenge: teaching dance online. "I wanted to choose to travel rather than get to a point where I was tired of doing it, but I had to do it because that's how I made my money. That's what transitioned me to online teaching—also the fact that I can reach more people this way."

The first challenge Andrew had to overcome was his fear that he needed to be with people physically in order to teach them how to dance. Over the last couple of years putting this practice to work through his Dance Ninjas training, he has discovered something interesting. "That is absolutely not true. It's actually quite easy to teach my students. The hard part is motivating them. How do you motivate someone to take the time to learn when it's not for a specific time, and there aren't people expecting them to show up? It has to be more about the value they're getting from the material, so you have to do a great job of explaining what they're going to get from each class. That's great, though, because it's improving my teaching skills in general and my sales skills as well."

In fact, it is through witnessing his sales and marketing skills that I know what Andrew is trying to teach his dance students extends far beyond dance. I asked him to elaborate on those side lessons, which made his eyes light up with passion and his words flow with extra vigor. "For me, the whole concept of learning dance communication is directly relatable to our regular lives. When we learn how to read if someone enjoys what we're doing or doesn't enjoy what we're doing, that is an extremely valuable bit of information that can transfer into other areas of our lives *so* strongly.

"We rely so much in the dance community on nonverbal communication that sometimes I have to bring people back to using verbal communication. I have to remind them that they *have* a voice and that they can speak to their partner and let them know what they enjoyed or didn't enjoy or why they want to dance right now or don't want to dance right now.

"My entire concept of fusion—of using your movement, your partner's movement, and the music together—has the fundamental goal of making every dance amazing. I don't want to go out to dance just to dance—I want to have amazing dances! I'm not going to succeed every time, but that's my goal. And then I think, what's my goal in life? It's to have an amazing life, to experience amazing things and have amazing interactions with everyone.

"There are so many times in dance where we sabotage ourselves. We get stuck in this mindset that a move is supposed to be done a certain way, and often it's because that's what we were taught. Then we go out with a partner, and they're not doing it that way, so we have this idea that they're not doing it right. That doesn't make the dance amazing! So a lot of my teaching is pointing out to people where they're doing that in their own dancing, because sometimes it's hard to see.

"It wasn't until many years after I'd been teaching this concept that I realized I was still doing this to my partners. The moment I realized that, I thought, 'How do I make the dance amazing if they *do* do that? Instead of complaining, how do I make that move amazing?' Only five minutes later, I had at least two ways of very clearly making it way better than ever before. What I find so amazing about that is all it took was asking one question and spending a few minutes thinking about it to provide me with hundreds of hours of more amazing dances.

"That's what I'm trying to teach people. To keep an open mind. And I believe it's the same in our lives. We have these ideas of how life has to be, how people need to communicate or live, when there are so many different ways of doing things and ways to make all those things amazing. Sometimes I don't know how to make it amazing; I just know that it's possible."

After all these years teaching, Andrew still considers himself an eager student—of both dance and life. "I'm constantly taking classes of all levels and from teachers with different mindsets. The more I can understand all these different ways of dancing, as well as just living life—when I travel to all these different cultures, I see ways of living that are completely different—the more I am able to help people and give examples of how others have been able to make different ways of teaching and living amazing."

I asked Andrew to give me an example of how what he has learned through dance has played out in his life. He didn't hesitate before sharing, "For me, the concept of fusion involves there being no wrong for my partner. I don't know if there's a wrong for me or not, I don't think of it in those terms. If I want to make an amazing dance, I have to find a way to make everything my partner does amazing.

"It's the same thing in relationships. There are times when everything my girlfriend says or does feels just *wrong*. But if I approach her in that way, we end up fighting. At some point, I realize I was not listening or communicating as effectively as I could have been; I'd been living in my tunnel vision, and when I can step out of that, we can have a much more beneficial conversation, one that takes us somewhere where we can learn from that disagreement.

"I look back fifteen years ago before I started dancing; my fights with my partner could last days or maybe even weeks. But after I understood and started practicing these concepts, days turned into hours and hours turned into minutes, and now I can sometimes catch myself before it even happens. In the last few years, the longest I can remember ever being mad at someone would have been a couple hours. It never lasts longer than that anymore. I imagine ten years from now, I'll be able to say the longest time I remember being mad was minutes. That's really one of the biggest things that the fusion mindset does for me."

I knew Andrew wasn't all talk; I had personally experienced him demonstrate these concepts with extreme success. He had taken a raw beginner, which I was back in 2007, and not only given me an amazing dance experience but given me the confidence and the inspiration to continue my pursuance of this dance. I left our interview feeling inspired yet again—to reach deeper within myself to find how I could offer more openness, more acceptance of both my dance and life partners. This is why I believe the healing of the planet can begin on the dance floor—and why Andrew has dedicated so much of himself to teaching these concepts to as many people as possible.

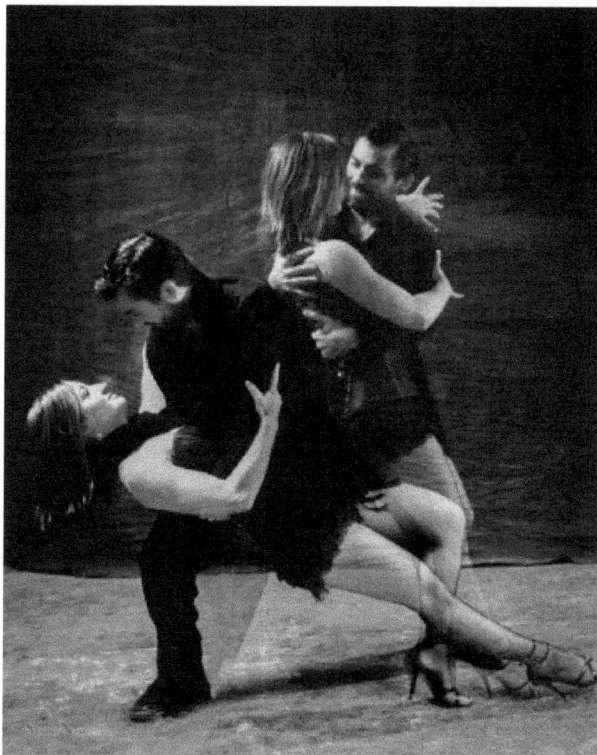

Photo by Samuel Nesbitt

II
BODY

Dance has been used as a form of therapy since early human history. Healing rituals took place to help overcome grief, prepare for birth, and recover from illness. Dance as a recognized form of physical and cognitive therapy, however, occurred relatively recently, in the 1950s. As a result of the work of American dancer and choreographer Marian Chase, dance movement therapy became an established modality within the medical community to aid in the recovery of motor skills and to serve as a psychotherapeutic tool for expressing emotions.

The styles of dance used in this medical movement are most often modern or ballroom dancing. What blues dancing offers is an additional layer of intimacy, vulnerability, and self-expression within a partnered connection. These added elements are what the stories in this book involve—but this section focuses on the healing of the body.

It can be difficult to distinguish between healing of the body and healing of the mind and spirit, the composite of which represents an individual's holistic well-being. But the following stories carry primary themes representative of health as it relates to awareness and rehabilitation of the physical body. Using dance in recovery from severe neurological conditions, muscular pain, and broken bones…using dance as a physical fitness program—here are six inspirational stories of individuals who have overcome significant obstacles by dancing to the blues.

Transforming the Most Difficult Relationship in My Life

Cara Bennett, Southampton, England

Most of us don't suspect our story is worthy of sharing—until someone else suggests that in fact it is. That's what happened with Cara. I made an announcement about this book at a dance event in London, calling for stories of transformation. A friend nudged her to participate, but she didn't feel comfortable declaring, "I have something to say." Several months later, however, Cara changed her mind. She realized she had something to say that could inspire people to improve their relationships with their bodies—and that was certainly a story worth sharing.

Cara's story of transformation began when she went from a "normal" nine-year-old kid growing up in Pittsburgh, Pennsylvania, to one with fibromyalgia and chronic fatigue syndrome. In attempting to describe what the condition has become for her, Cara explained, "Every inch of my body is in pain every second of every day. My muscles, my joints, my insides, my outsides…even my eyelids hurt. Then there's the fatigue. Imagine twenty years of sleep deprivation with no reprieve—it's called 'nonrestorative sleep.' Unsurprisingly, chronic depression goes along with the chronic fatigue."

To say Cara's relationship with her body is fraught is to put it lightly. "My body is the source of all my pain and 'failures.' It has forced me to sacrifice a career, the possibility of having children, and countless interests, hobbies, and relationships. The pain and fatigue makes experiencing joy almost impossible at times." By the time Cara turned eighteen, she was so sick, she couldn't get out of bed.

Unfortunately, there is no cure for her condition; there is only managing the pain and fatigue. So Cara has dedicated herself to studying health and wellness in an effort to do just that, for herself and for others.

"I educated myself about nutrition and learned that the three things that help manage my health are the same for the average person—getting sleep, exercising, and eating healthy. So I started exercising for the first time since I was fourteen. If I don't exercise for a day, my pain levels go up, which generally makes it more difficult to sleep. I had participated in gymnastics, soccer, and tennis. But when I quit sports, my health got so much worse. I never put the two together—that stopping exercise would actually make me *more* tired."

The suggestion that exercise would ease her pain and fatigue seemed counterintuitive to her for years, until she began researching the topic. "I was stunned by the weight of scientific evidence that shows exercise helps pain, sleep, alertness and mood. What exercise does is address the imbalance in neurotransmitters, which is both a cause and an effect of my sleep deprivation and depression. Neurotransmitters help us regulate sleep, but certain neurotransmitters and hormones, including endorphins and adrenaline, also kill pain and enhance mood."

As a university student, she began incorporating solo dancing into her exercise routine. "I'd go out club dancing three nights a week, every single week. The high that I got from it was incredible; dancing sweated out the pain. Even though I'd only have had three hours of sleep the night before, that euphoria carried me through the next day. Dancing is what got me through university. I'd tell myself, if I can just get through the next few days, I can go out dancing again."

That was Cara's first experience with the joy that she felt through dancing. She didn't discover partner dancing until after college, when she moved to Ithaca, New York, with her husband. The two of them signed up for Lindy Hop classes. Lindy Hop gave her the exercise high that she craved, but when she discovered blues dancing four or five months later—a discovery that often evolves from first having learned the jazz steps of Lindy Hop—she fell in love.

Five years later, she's still dancing to the blues. She has good reason to continue. "Blues dancing—and exercise in general—is a chance for me to do something positive with my body. When I dance, my body is not only the source of joy and pleasure—it is the conduit for that joy and pleasure. I stop growling at my body and instead start thanking my body for allowing me to express myself and to connect with others in a completely unique and intangible way. By the end of a night when the endorphins are flowing, I feel immensely proud and empowered that I have found a way to transform the most difficult relationship in my life."

I was beginning to learn how Cara's healing through dance extends far beyond reprieve from pain. "There are so many ways blues dancing has impacted and improved my relationship with my body. I get an endorphin rush from the exercise, I feel alive and joyful from the music, and then I have the experience of connection with others. Human contact is so powerful. There is such healing power in touch, and I feel like a lot of people miss out on that."

Cara does not look solely to dance to fulfill that need for human connection and physical intimacy. She is grateful to have an understanding and supportive husband. She admits that having a partner who is chronically ill, depressed, and unable to work full-time can put a lot of pressure on a relationship, but her marriage remains strong despite those challenges.

"I'm blessed with a partner who makes sure I never feel like an emotional or financial burden and who creates a safe space for me to be myself, even if that means being angry or depressed." Though it may mean she has to work less or see him less, he also encourages her love of dancing. "He knows how restorative it is for my body and soul. I always come home from a festival full of good vibes."

Though dancing has significantly improved her health, she still struggles with the symptoms of her condition. Although she's an advocate for encouraging more movement into people's lives, she does not pretend that dance—or exercise in general—is a cure-all for those with chronic conditions such as hers. "Fatigue and depression are still big issues for me. The pain makes sleeping or staying in the present moment difficult, but it is not as disabling as the exhaustion. It's the fatigue that actually changes who you are—it actually takes away your identity. When I dance, I feel like myself for a bit. The best version of myself. I feel alive, connected to the world, and unlimited.

"I've spent years trying to distract myself from my body and from the pain inside of me. When I started dancing, instead of running from my body, I found pleasure and joy from *using* my body. I started to realize early on that I was doing something incredibly therapeutic.

"Exercise first changed my life—I love working out. But dancing was therapeutic in a completely different way. My body was *giving* me joy. When I'm dancing, my body is the source of everything good in that moment. I feel so alive when I dance; I feel tingly and otherworldly. It's beyond the physical; it feels spiritual. I don't practice a particular faith or spirituality, but I don't know how to describe it without that word. How do you describe that feeling to someone that hasn't had that experience?"

Cara's gaze moved from her webcam, through which we were speaking, to somewhere far off in the distance. I could feel her reliving her most memorable moments on the dance floor as she continued. "That four hours—or even thirty minutes—of deep transcendence that happens when dancing...It is something that comes from really deep inside of you. It's not something that is happening *to* you—you are creating it. I'm not thinking about pain. I'm not thinking at all!"

When I asked her how dance fits into her daily routine, she replied, "I now incorporate dance more and more into my life; I always enjoy putting on music and dancing at home, but I do it more intentionally now. I build it into my workouts; I make a point to dance. There are days when I'm feeling so weak and so low, and I know that I'll feel better if I work out, but *god*, I don't feel like it.

"Finally, I just say, okay, I'll put a song on and just see what happens. I play some music and move around a little bit, and I find that it makes me smile, and I start dancing, and I suddenly come alive. My body *creates* energy. The lethargy is completely gone, because my body is actually creating energy and joy, and that's helped me so many times to just get started with my day."

As I said, Cara almost didn't share her story. But what convinced her to open up was her desire to share this particular message: "If you're depressed or feeling down in any way, there are so many studies that show that releasing endorphins and adrenaline helps. Add the additional layer of connection to others, connection to music, and self-expression, and it can transform the way that you relate to your body. You can discover emotional and physical sensations that you never knew were there; you can start to *want* to interact with your body, instead of running away from it. Dancing is a tool that can help you see your body in a positive way. Your body can do amazing things, it can feel amazing things, it can create sensations that change your entire worldview."

To hear those words from someone whose body and life opportunities have been compromised as much as hers, it's hard not to take that message to heart. It's a reminder that she herself needs to hear sometimes.

"I can be so depressed at times, when I genuinely don't believe that my life is worth living. And yet when I'm dancing, when I'm experiencing that transcendental joy, I feel so alive. I *want* to be alive! In those moments, I feel like life really does have something to offer, even for me. I'm not sure if I'm going to be alive at ninety years old, but if I am alive, I really hope I'm dancing."

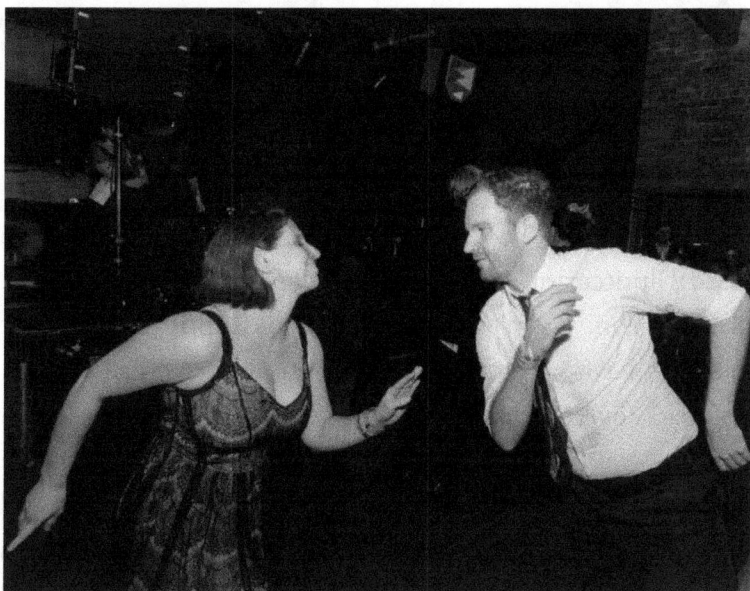

Photo by mswheelerphotography

Dancing with Your Breath…and a Broken Leg

Eros Salvatore, Port Townsend, Washington, USA

Life is full of serendipity. I met Eros while volunteering at a Blues Recess event in northern Washington. It was rainy and cold, but that didn't dampen Eros's spirits, even though he looked as though he had every reason to be something other than happy—he was at a dance event with a broken leg! He hobbled on crutches to the outdoor registration tent and sat down next to me to wait for the event organizer's return to help him with a question that only she could answer. He was told it could be an hour, but he didn't mind the wait.

In most new social situations, people in our culture typically begin getting to know each other with the question, "So, what do you do?" Not the case with dancers. I began by asking Eros, "So, how did you first get involved in the dance scene?" That led to the story of Eros's life as seen through the lens of dance—a much more interesting tale than the former question usually generates. He did not come to me with the expectation of being interviewed for a book, but it makes perfect sense in retrospect. He was born to a writer, and knows a story can be unearthed at any given moment—anywhere.

"I was born in a small town in Ireland where my dad went to write a book. The book was about a town that was very alternative and thought that it was the center of the universe. I was conceived and born in that town, and my whole life I've lived in different alternative towns or communities that feel like the center of the universe. Blues Recess is one of those communities." Eros laughed. I agreed. The event got its name from its mission to provide a "recess" from traditional norms and constructions. The location we were at—like the locations of most Blues Recess events—was "off the grid," offering the sense of isolation from the rest of the world.

Eros learned to blues dance in Seattle about twelve years ago, after becoming familiar with swing dancing. "One night, I was feeling very depressed and alone, and I went for a walk. I was walking down Eighty-Fifth Avenue and Greenwood, and I looked up, and I saw these lights in the window on the second floor. I heard swing music, and I thought, 'Wow, that sounds amazing!' I thought it was a restaurant, and I went behind back to check it out. I walked up the stairs, and there were a bunch of people dancing. I asked the people at the door, 'What is this?!' And they told me, 'It's swing dancing; we do this every week.' I asked if I could sit down, and they welcomed me in."

But if there is a shortage of males, one does not sit on the dance floor sidelines for long. "Soon after I sat down, this beautiful girl comes up and asks me to dance. I told her I didn't know how to dance, and she said, 'That doesn't matter! I'll show you.' We danced, and from there I immediately became involved in the

East Coast swing dance scene, then right into blues and the whole blues fusion scene that was just starting to develop."

Eros's first experience with blues dancing was at an underground blues dance in Capitol Hill in Seattle. "I went down to this basement room, and it was really warm and sweaty. I attended the lesson, and it was so easy. That was the thing that I loved about it—I had been doing swing dancing, which required learning multiple steps and moves, but blues dancing can be learned without ever having done a partner dance before. So I fell in love with it. I'd always loved blues music, the old traditional blues stuff. I used to play guitar and was into Robert Johnson, and one of his songs came on at the dance, so it came full circle."

Eros would soon move away from Seattle, to a series of small towns and cities that did not have blues dancing. When he returned to Seattle for a visit nearly ten years later, he stopped by a venue he used to dance at, which happened to be hosting a fusion dance that night. He immediately loved this style—a blend of blues, sometimes swing, and any other form of creative movement the dancer may use to self-express—and ended up striking up conversation with attendees who were from Port Townsend, a small town a couple of hours northwest and, interestingly, where he was about to move to. They shared that although the town was small, there was a fusion dance community there.

"That is where I got really into fusion dancing. It became a very powerful and enjoyable part of my life and made me connect with people physically like I'd never been able to do before."

It was through the fusion community there that he learned about the Blues Recess event, outside of which we now sat, during this impromptu interview. He almost didn't make it, however. "I was so excited about coming to this event, but then I broke my leg last month. I didn't think I'd be able to come, which was unfortunate because I live just across Puget Sound." It was also his birthday the day of his arrival, so to stay home would have been disappointing for more than one reason.

Often for events such as this, the dance community posts an online ride-share board. Eros couldn't drive with his broken leg, so he checked the board on the off chance that someone from his small town had listed there. Much to his surprise, a guy flying a two-seater 150 Cessna plane to the event was looking for a passenger. Eros described the experience: "We took off at 8:00 p.m. on Monday night with a full moon from Port Townsend, and we buzzed over Seattle. We watched the Mariners play baseball, and we saw Seattle and the Space Needle become tiny, and it was just so beautiful. We were in this plane at one hundred miles an hour, and nobody was around us. I thought, 'Everyone should be up here on a Saturday night! This is what we should *all* be doing.'" He laughed.

"I've had this amazing, serendipitous experience here. It's been very healing for me; the people here are so welcoming and helpful. It's the best broken-leg dance event you could have."

When I asked what he thought his life would be like without dancing, Eros had a ready answer. "I would be lost. I would be stumbling, as I am now on my broken leg. Life would be very depressing and tragic without dancing. It's what keeps me going."

This wasn't the first occasion Eros had needed—and received—support from his fellow dancers due to a physical challenge. "I've had a series of physical problems over the past several years. My arms were paralyzed a year and a half ago, so I couldn't use a computer or anything, and I developed emphysema and a bunch of other internal diseases that caused me to not be able to work. The dance community has always been there for me."

In Eros's opinion, dance can provide more than individual healing. "I believe that dancing can change the world. Everybody needs to dance. It's part of the human spirit. The culture has chopped itself up so much that a lot of it is isolated; different cultures isolate themselves within themselves, so you have pockets of people who don't dance or do anything in community."

And why limit dancing to only those who can walk? As the contributors to this section reveal, there are ways to work around perceived limitations. "Even with a broken leg, I've experimented with dancing a few times. Even if I was in a wheelchair, I could dance. There's always some rhythm and movement going on inside of us. If you can feel the breath in your body, there's a rhythm to that. The blood beating through your heart is like a beat that goes on. There's actually dancing inside of you all the time. You can't actually live without it."

I couldn't have said it better myself. It's no surprise Eros comes from a family of writers.

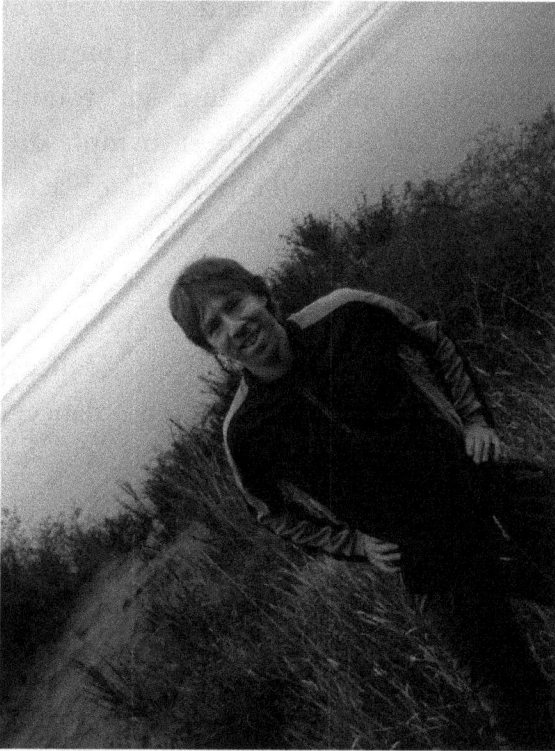

Dancing Is My Fitness Program

Anna Takkula, Newcastle upon Tyne, England

There are many versions of Anna. I danced with two of them while attending a four-day dance event in the summer of 2014 called the European Blues Invasion (EBI), held in London, England. One version was a seemingly quiet sixty-five-year-old Finnish woman casually dressed in jeans, a T-shirt, and round glasses. The other was an ethereal forest nymph dressed in green tights with fringe at the bottom, a black top hat, and large pointed ears. I didn't realize the two women were actually the same person until after the latter dance had ended and she'd removed her hat and ears.

The theme of that particular dance was A Midsummer Night's Dream, and dancers were encouraged to dress accordingly. That is a suggestion Anna never takes lightly. I have since seen photos of Anna in extravagant ballroom, 1920s speakeasy, and formal masquerade dance attire. When I later caught up with Anna for this interview, I had to ask her what inspires her to participate so passionately in costume contests.

Anna laughed joyfully, and her eyes lit up in pride and amusement as she replied, "I don't know! What happened this time [for EBI] is I went into this costume sale earlier in the summer, and I found what was the basis for my costume: the leggings. I was sure someday I'd find them useful. So when I heard the theme was A Midsummer Night's Dream, I thought, 'Yes! I'm going to go all out for this one!' I guess I'm a bit theatrical; two of my boys are actors, so perhaps they got some of that from me. I'm not an actor, but there must be something of it in me."

Dressing in elaborate costumes was not the only quality I found unique about Anna. I often saw her leading blues more often than following—which, although it is a growing phenomenon among women in the blues dance scene, is still rather uncommon. I was unaccustomed enough to this circumstance that I was surprised when Anna first asked me to dance, not long after meeting her as a fellow volunteer at EBI. What I was even more surprised to discover, however, was just how *good* the dance felt. Anna's technique was playful and creative, and her dance frame was more solid than that of many men I had danced with earlier in the night. I could tell she'd been doing this a while, and she later revealed how her journey as a dance lead began.

"It was with salsa dancing. I had just started taking lessons and going to the dances afterward. I looked at the huge number of women sitting there, and I thought, 'I didn't come here to sit! The only way I can do more dancing is by leading, so then I will lead.' The sheer frustration of not wanting to go to a dance and just sit around was enough motivation for me. I was a total beginner as a follow, so I was a total beginner as a lead as well. I would go to the beginner lessons, and I would lead or follow depending on who was there.

"Now I lead blues too. Leading blues is as amazing as following blues. I really recommend it. It's different with blues than it is with salsa, and especially with microblues, which is much more intimate. I had a surprising experience with one woman once. I danced microblues with a man, and this woman saw me. She said it was amazing to watch, and though she was about to leave, she asked me if the next time we were at the dance, if I would lead her. I'm totally heterosexual, and I'm thinking, 'How is *that* going to work?'

"Anyway, a promise is a promise, so at the next blues dance, I led her in microblues for a whole song, and it was completely fine. It just felt really good. At the end of the song, she was like, 'That was really deep and so invigorating!' and that was such an amazing realization for me, that it really is fine to dance so intimately with a woman. It just works on so many levels; blues dancing has really given me a lot more freedom in partner dancing and in using different parts of my body and enjoying physical movement and closeness with people. I haven't been in a relationship for over a year now, and I don't really miss it. I am getting a lot of hugs and physical closeness through dance, and specifically through blues dancing."

Leading has revealed other things to Anna about herself too. "It's really weird, all the obnoxious stuff that comes in your head when you lead. When you're following, you're really not worried about doing a lot of moves, but then when you start leading, you think, 'I wonder if she's bored. I wonder if I should start throwing this big move in. What move can I do?'"

Anna has a trick to get out of her head and back into the dance, however. "I first and foremost connect with the music. Especially with blues, I feel the music inside of me. It gives me a connection with my partner that is physical, but there's also a shared connection because we're listening to the same music. Very seldom am I aware of anything or anybody else in the room when I dance, so I'm very much dancing with that one person. The weird thing is especially when I follow, I can almost read the lead's mind and know whether they're thinking about the music or about the next move. There's a difference between the quality of dancing when the lead is concentrating on what they should do next or when they are considering the music. Guess which one is better." Anna grinned.

Anna's mythical experience isn't limited only to her costume at EBI—she has had dances that felt otherworldly as well. "I had quite an incredible experience. I was dancing switch dancing, where we trade who is leading and following, and it was after we'd taken these classes about expressing different tempos in different parts of your body. So in the last minute of the song while switch dancing with this guy in close embrace, I tried doing fast shimmies with my body while moving slowly with my feet and the lead was just like, 'How did you *do* that?! That was amazing!' He was completely, positively thrown. It was a brilliant experience for me that my leading could have that kind of impact on somebody. I've had moments while dancing blues when the world could have exploded and blown to pieces, and I wouldn't have known it because the dance was just so connected."

I was curious how often Anna goes out dancing. To have reached her level, she must go out frequently, I assumed, but her answer surprised me.

"When I'm at home in Newcastle, I try not to dance on Wednesdays." Anna paused and held a mischievous smile, waiting to see if I understood the nuance. She could see I did not, so she laughed and explained, "That means that the six other days of the week, I dance." This was a feat I found incredible; it's often physically unattainable even for people in their twenties or thirties, and I felt my admiration for this woman increase exponentially.

"When I go to dance conferences, I do the lessons, and then I go eat a pasta meal to get energy, and then I sleep, and then I return to the dance at about ten or eleven at night. So, often I don't take part in the first part of the dance or the competitions, so I can sleep while that is on, and then I go for the dancing afterward. I try to organize my time so I don't burn out, because I can't do twenty-four hours."

I don't know anyone who can, I thought, but if anyone could—Anna would be a good contestant.

"Dancing is my fitness program. It is the running theme in my life; I don't do it to keep fit—I do it so I can dance better. But it keeps me fit. Dancing made me realize I need more balance and stronger core muscles, so that led me to do Pilates. Because of dancing, I have also had to pay attention to my posture, and it has improved over the years too.

"It has even changed the way I buy clothes. Most of the time I go to the shop, and I think, 'Can I dance in this one?'" Anna once again laughed with amusement at her own behavior.

"One of the regrets I do have is that I was over forty when I got into dancing. It would have been really nice to have done it earlier. But at the same time, I'm glad I did it when I did; it's something that any age person can do and with any level of physical ability. One of the things I've started doing is wheelchair dancing, and that has just blown my mind. I have not found a place in England yet to do that, but at the group I go to in Finland, the whole point is that everybody can and will dance. It doesn't matter what level of disability you have. They always think, 'Okay, we're doing this move, but you can do it this way, or you can do it that way. Let's see what way you can do this dance.'

"That's really revolutionary for my thinking, the fact that everybody can move somehow, and it's not that I have to make people do the move the way I want. I may have to change the move so that the person can do it to their ability. I don't know anyone who does blues dancing in wheelchairs, so I bought myself a wheelchair, and I'm going to start trying to figure out how to dance blues in a wheelchair."

Anna will tell you that dancing has brought many wonderful and unexpected experiences into her life.

"Before coming to EBI, one of my friends said, 'You need to make a treasure map—putting down things that you want in life—and in a very surprising way, they will happen.' So I sent her this email of three things I really wanted in my life, and one of them was that I want to go to a Blues Recess event in the United States.

"This was like three days before EBI, and the organizer of the Blues Recess events was there at EBI, so I thought I would talk to him and see if I could go to an event for free by working for it. Well, I never had a chance to talk to him, but I won the costume competition, which was a free pass to a Blues Recess event! Dreams can come through in many surprising ways."

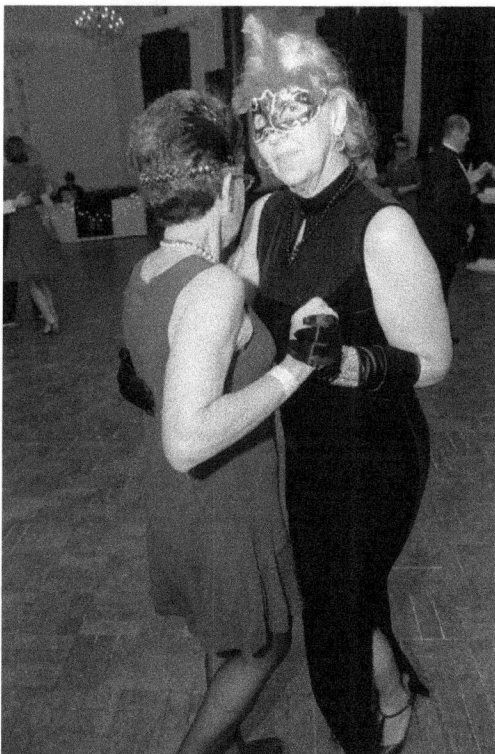

Photo by Jason Roseweir

Back Pain and the Beauty of the Present Moment

Ian Burke, London, England

I remember the first time I saw Ian walk into a room. He was tall and lithe, with a presence that made me pay attention. We were at a dance in London. Until then, I had had few inspiring dances—which was probably due to my own insecurities—and I was considering leaving early. But instead, I watched Ian begin to dance with a woman I also could not take my eyes off of. They clearly had chemistry, but it wasn't just their chemistry that drew me in. It was their *style*. I'd never seen anything quite like it. They took up a lot of space, incorporating many dips and what I can only describe as controlled whips: I could see the flow of energy generated from a particular body part of his—a shoulder, for example—that would then spread in a wave down the arm, through the wrist, and out the fingertips until it took possession of his partner's own body. I could already feel how my experience of the night was about to shift.

I don't believe Ian would have noticed me; I did not carry much of a presence of my own that night, so I took it upon myself to catch him for a dance before anyone else could. What happened was magic—it was one of those dances that is so intense that at the song's closing note, there is a silent, mutual understanding that the embrace will not be released but will instead extend into the next song.

That was my introduction to Ian …although I wouldn't even find out his name until a couple of weeks later, when a crowdfunding promotion passed through my Facebook feed. He turned out to be a filmmaker, working on a documentary about the transformational power of partner dancing. I immediately recognized the opportunity to collaborate. And so it was that I officially introduced myself at the next dance event we both attended—the European Blues Invasion (EBI)—where I came to learn more about the film project he was working on with Claire Loussouan (the woman I had seen him dancing with that first night). Our projects were in such alignment that I ended up sharing my story in his film—and now his is one of the stories in my book. It was only as a result of this interview that I learned there was a significant time period in Ian's adult life when he couldn't even walk properly, let alone dance.

Ian began dancing at a fairly young age. "It was something I secretly liked to do, but it just wasn't that hip." It was the post-punk era in London at the time; there was no partner dance culture as it exists today, he shared. However, there was an active club scene of which Ian actively took part. He was working as a professional musician at the time, so his lifestyle was already a late-night one.

His musicianship lasted for about ten years. After playing in crowded pubs five or six nights a week, without paying any attention to the ergonomics of how he was playing, coupled with going out dancing after each gig and ignoring his body then too, Ian developed repetitive strain injury in his hands and arms. The pain grew so massive that he had to stop playing.

But he continued going out partying and dancing all night. At some point, however, he came home and noticed that his back really hurt. "I'd have to lay down for a bit. I didn't really think too much of it, but after a while it got really bad; my back would go into spasm, and it would take a few days to recover. It dawned on me that whatever was going on was getting quite serious, but I didn't think there was something in my dancing that was creating the back problem." He continued dancing, until the spasms got longer and longer, and eventually the pain became constant, and he couldn't even walk properly.

He never gave up dancing, though. For a year and a half, he walked with a stick that opens up to a little seat. "Whenever I went to festivals and parties, I'd take that stick. I'd sit on the stick, and I could dance around without actually standing up. It was my way of still being able to go out and interact; I could be social and dance in my own funny sort of way."

But after about six months of that, Ian started to get really depressed. "I got into this mindset that I might always be like that. I had to rethink my life completely. I might not be able to run; I'll have to watch how I walk—so anything like trekking or taking long walks was completely out of the question. I could walk down to the shops, so I wasn't completely immobile, but I was definitely a bit of an invalid."

What caused Ian to go off the deep end wasn't his body as much as his mind. "I got into this mindset that I *am* that person, and that's when I started to get depressed. The one thing that I could really pinpoint as the source of identifying with being an invalid was my inability to dance. That's when I realized how important dance had become to me."

As it is for so many people, Ian finds dance cathartic. Dancing is his way of "putting himself out into the world." Not having that form of self-expression made him anxious and affected his state of mind, so he was inspired to do some research. "I read a book about back pain, and it said that the worst thing you can do for muscular pain—which most back pain is—was to ponder to it. Don't start to identify with it, just work through it—which was the opposite of what I was doing. I was like, 'Oh, I've got pain; don't put any stress on that side of my body,' and I'd start walking around a little funny just so I wouldn't make any jerky movements."

Ian was already doing Pilates to try to rehabilitate, and once he got to the point where he could start to move a bit, he started practicing tai chi and yoga. But he still missed dancing. Rather than club dancing, however, a woman he was dating suggested he try tango. "I liked the idea of tango because it was almost like doing tai chi with a partner. It's going back to the basics and just walking around the room, but being really mindful of your walking. I thought, well, that's the sort of thing I need to do—I need to relearn how to walk, how to move on a very basic level."

During the first couple of months out dancing again—tango and, later, swing dancing—he feared he would injure himself beyond repair. But he kept coming back to the idea that he shouldn't cater to the pain but, rather, work through it. He still experienced pain after each class, but he noticed it hadn't gotten worse, so he kept going. Eventually, he noticed it was actually getting better; he was able to incorporate more movements into his dancing. "In the beginning, I'd have to sit down after a few dances and then get up and try again. But after two weeks of just hitting the basics, it felt amazing to be able to dance again. After two years of thinking of myself as an invalid who couldn't move anymore, it was just so revelatory."Ian was hooked. Not so much on tango and swing dancing but on movement. He still tried to keep from overdoing it, but he found that he could increase the number of nights he went out dancing to sometimes even five nights a week. It didn't take long for his depression to fall away; he instantly noticed the connection between movement and not just physical health but mental health. It even altered the way he thought about gender roles.

"Once I started partner dancing, I gained a new perspective on the physical role of a man. I came of age in the '80s, and in England it was a time of political correctness with gender. Partner dancing almost became bad taste as a guy, because to play the role of the lead—

to have control over the woman—was seen as disrespectful. It was almost to the point where you don't want to exhibit masculinity even, because it's too forceful."

This new awareness of his ingrained beliefs and fears regarding his role as a man would become deeper questioned once he became involved with the blues dance community. It wasn't until he attended a blues dance event that he realized what he'd been dancing more closely resembled the modern blues dance aesthetic. "I can't remember how I ended up at the dance, but I walked in and saw how they were dancing and thought, 'Oh! They've got a name for it!' As far as I could gather, they were improvising in a close embrace dance. I always liked that close embrace from tango, but I loved that this dance didn't have any particular steps to it."

Around the same time, a friend of his invited him to the first European Blues Invasion dance event in London in 2012. He decided to attend, and it didn't take long for him to discover that the style of blues this event emphasized—which was "alternative blues," or "fusion"—was where his heart lies.

"I took a few classes at EBI and watched some of the jams, and I was like, 'That is it!' That is how I dance, taken up a notch. The way they were interacting was really gender fluid, and I started to make the connection, that, okay, there's this dance, but there's also a bit of a lifestyle behind this dancing that doesn't exist in London, but it seems to exist with some of these

American people." The lifestyle Ian was referring to was what modern culture would call "alternative"—one without rules or enforced conformity, which is the celebrated lifestyle at Blues Recess events.

Ian was so inspired by what he was observing and experiencing within the blues fusion dance community that he became enthralled with the idea of merging his two passions in life—dancing and filmmaking. "I've done a lot of filming around dancing over the years; it's just an aesthetically beautiful thing to see." Now, however, he wanted to go beyond filming dance to filming a documentary that explored the connections among dance, gender roles, and alternative lifestyles and relationships. He discussed it with Claire, who has a background in anthropology and used to go to dance parties with Ian. He figured she'd be on board with the project.

She was. And so was Justin Riley, one of the organizers of the European Blues Invasion. Ian sat down with him for an interview, where he got the inside scoop on the Blues Recess scene, as well as how fusion dancing was kicking off in America and becoming its own lifestyle.

He decided to go see it for himself. Ian recognized that it was key to come to the United States for filming, where the lead-follow seems to fluctuate. "To me, this switch culture that's happening in the blues dance scene demonstrates how society has gotten to a more mature place with gender and sexual polarity in dance."

Ian and Claire flew to the United States for a Blues Recess event near Aspen, Colorado, followed by another Blues Recess event near Bellingham, Washington, in the summer of 2014. To get the full experience, the two rode with the organizers on the Recess Bus from one event to the next. "On the bus we filmed these moments of reflection about time and the idea of constant motion and impermanence—the idea that a dance is fleeting and the inherent beauty in the fact that it is fleeting."

To Ian, dance is a metaphor for being in the present moment. "A dance is so short-lived it forces you to appreciate the present moment. Chasing after permanence almost forces you out of the present moment. Leading and following is like talking and listening at the same time. As leads we have a tendency to anticipate the next moment but blues promotes a listening culture of allowing each moment to unfold based on the dynamics of the bodies involved and the surrounding dance floor. It becomes a mindfulness exercise—a meditation—in its own right."

Another takeaway from his experience in the US alternative blues scene is that intimacy can be experienced outside of the normal cultural paradigms that it's set in. "That's something I want to demonstrate in the film—this idea that we can experience intimacy with anybody. I think a lot of people crave the experience of intimacy outside the confines of one particular partner or relationship. What partner dancing does is give us what we crave in a way that is socially acceptable."

What Ian feels makes blues dancing more intimate than other dances is the fact that it has no steps or structure. "You're forced to improvise, which makes you very vulnerable. I think that's what puts people off more than the physical closeness—the fact that you're just out there with somebody, and nobody's really told you what to do. You have to find a way to interact with each other and the music."

Ian points out that the music doesn't necessarily tell you what to do either. "Dancing to music that has space is what defines this type of dance for me. There are not many dance forms that specifically seek out spacious music, because it doesn't tell you what to do. That is what blues music does so well; it's minimalist music in a way. I like the old, early acoustic blues, which has very little in it, just beautiful musicianship that's almost ambient in the way it's played."

Not being told what to do is, I believe, what makes Ian such a pleasure to dance with. Whatever insecurities I had that first night I saw him fell away the moment we began dancing together—without using words, he communicated to me that anything goes. I think that's the ultimate gift we can offer another: total acceptance of how our partner shows up. In fact, that's the best gift we can offer ourselves too.

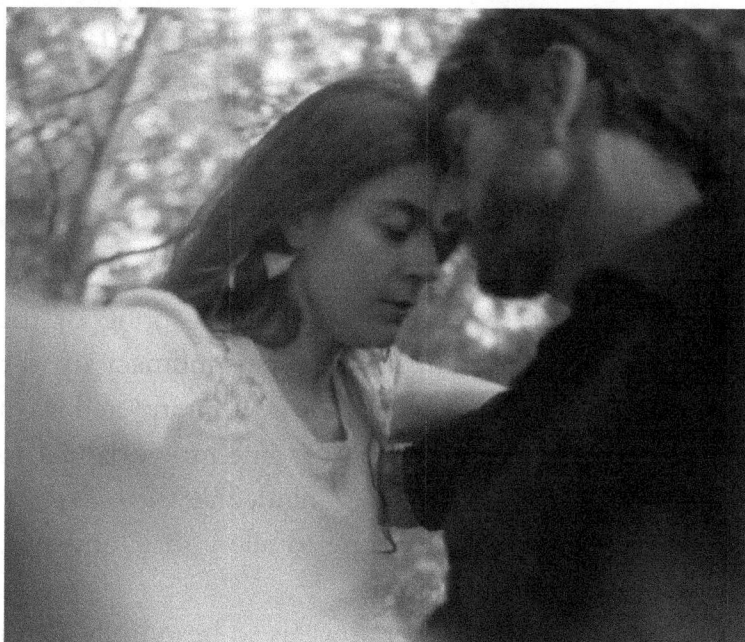

Expressing on the Outside What I Feel on the Inside

Alyx LeBeau, Vancouver, British Columbia, Canada

To the casual observer of a blues dance—someone who is not so familiar with or accepting of the distinction between intimacy on versus intimacy off the dance floor—blues dancing is often interpreted as a sexual dance. It's hard for even some grown adults to find the courage—or the open-mindedness—to explore the dance themselves, let alone to allow their underage children to participate in it.

But what Alyx's story reveals so beautifully about the modern blues dance scene is that you can gain valuable adult lessons from the dance and its community without compromising what society labels as "appropriate" young adult behavior. In fact, it may even dissuade youth from participating in the very behavior their parents would prefer they'd avoid, by offering a healthy outlet for teenage hormones and angst.

Alyx was in high school when she began blues dancing. She'd always had a passion for dance, but it wasn't something that was taught in her school. Her friend tried to teach her what she knew about dance, but it wasn't met with a positive result.

"As a teenager, I had a friend who was competing in solo dance competitions in hip-hop, jazz, and modern. She was training to be an instructor, and she started trying to teach me how to do certain moves. She eventually got frustrated and threw her hands up and said, 'I can't do this; you can't dance. You're not teachable.' I was like, 'Oh. Okay.' So for a long time I just thought I couldn't dance, but it never stopped me from wanting to."

Ever since she was a child, music has connected directly to Alyx's soul. "Dancing has given me the technique and the skill to be able to interpret the music—to finally be able to express on the outside what it feels like on the inside—and that's been incredibly liberating."

Like many people, she started blues dancing through Lindy Hop. One summer she was hanging out with a girlfriend of hers who for months had been telling her that she needed to go to a swing dancing event. She always replied, "No, no, no, it's not really my thing; my friends have told me I can't dance. I have no sense of balance, two left feet, et cetera." However, her friend knew Alyx needed a ride home that night, so she said, "I'll give you a ride home, but you have to come dancing first."

Alyx finally acquiesced. She ended up going to a Lindy Hop dance that was on a stage at the beach. There was no group class offered before this particular dance, so the organizer taught her as much as he could about Lindy Hop in twenty minutes. Alyx was surprised that this particular teacher did not consider her "unteachable," and she did pick up the rhythm and steps rather naturally. After experiencing the appeal of dancing—and the revelation that maybe she *could* dance— she continued to attend Lindy Hop events for a few months, until the organizer advertised a traditional blues dance event. Alyx attended, and from that night on, blues dancing had her heart.

"I got hooked on blues dancing much faster than I did on Lindy Hop. It was really hard as a new follow to get into the Lindy Hop scene because no one approached new people. If you're not confident in yourself, you're not going to get any dances. But with blues it was different. People were more approachable, I guess because of the intimate nature of the dance."

Alyx has been blues dancing for over seven years now, but she's had to take some breaks. At one point, she started experiencing really bad knee problems. She had to quit Lindy Hop completely because she had torn her ACL and meniscus, and it would lock up once or twice a month. She almost had to quit dancing entirely—but even when she couldn't dance, she stayed involved in the community. "I was part of a team that started up the first blues fusion event ever in Vancouver. It was a great transition period for me because I had the knee injury and couldn't dance, but it kept me involved in the scene until my knees started getting better. Sitting on the sidelines, I got to see firsthand what dancing can do for a person's well-being."

Alyx loved organizing and felt good to be able to provide something to the community. At an age when social pressure to go out drinking and partying was rampant, she took comfort in not only having an outlet to be social in a more constructive way but being able to offer others that opportunity. What many people who are new to the blues or swing dance scenes are surprised to discover is that social dances usually do not sell alcohol. The beverage of choice for most dancers in these communities is water—and a lot of it. Alyx was delighted, therefore, to play a part in expanding the awareness among her peers that dance venues existed as a worthy alternative to underage parties. "It was incredible to see how happy people were. I'd watch them come in, connect with others, dance, and then leave with smiles on their faces. How could you *not* want to do this?" Years later, Alyx is still helping grow the dance scene in Vancouver; she's currently co-organizing a weekly blues and fusion event that brings in instructors from the United States.

Only in the past year did she start figuring out how to manage her knee pain. "Before, I couldn't dance unless I was with very specific partners. I had to have very calm dances; I couldn't go over the top with it at all. I connected with dancers who have had similar injuries, who knew how to cater the dance so I wouldn't be injured. Even then, I'd have a maximum of five dances a night over four hours, before having to go home to ice my knee and take pain killers. But I'm in a much better place now."

Thanks to a dance class she took at a blues dance event in Portland, Oregon, last year, she had an epiphany. "It was a class on body mechanics and the fundamentals of blues and posture. I learned that below your core you've got this strip of muscle that's above your pelvis, and you have to angle your hips properly, so you're actually engaging the right leg muscles. We also learned about undulations. By identifying the muscles used in a body roll movement, I was able to know what it feels like to have proper posture."

In the class, each student worked with another to identify how to keep the spine straight, with all the vertebrae stacked upon each other—shoulders over hips over knees—bringing awareness to what was happening to the joints and the bones when using each one. Alyx was able to learn what she was doing right and what she was doing wrong, and, therefore, uncover what could be causing the pain. Once she established proper posture on a regular basis, she stopped having crippling back and knee pain. "I had woken up in pain every day before that, but with proper posture, the pain disappeared."

Alyx got emotional when she talked about the difference dance and body awareness has made in her life, "I've spent so many years not being able to do things. I now finally have this release. I've learned so much through dance that pain is almost nonexistent. It gets me choked up when I talk about it."

Her gratitude extends beyond the relief from pain to a general sense of acceptance of her injury and the opportunities that resulted from it. "Going to dance events, especially when there's a live band, and not being able to dance is absolute torture, but it allowed me to hone my social skills. I learned how to have conversations with people beyond the pleasantries of 'Hey, how are you doing? How's your day?'" Instead, she'd be encouraged to talk about careers, or dreams or fears. "I became able to interact with people from all different walks of life. In the blues scene, you get students, you get artists, you get your medium-income earners and your high-income earners. I was just coming into being an adult myself, so learning how to interact with adults was a big deal for me."

Like with any new skill, she first had to get over the fear of being new at something. "When I first started going to dances, it was nerve-racking. I didn't know how to put myself out there; I saw all these people who knew each other, who were really well connected, who were a lot older than me, so my initial reaction was that I don't fit in." But it was the very fact that she *was* so young that led people to notice her—and in turn make more of an effort to make her feel welcome.

Alyx didn't just learn how to communicate on a basic level with others—she learned how to express her feelings and thoughts on a deeper level than she could with her school-age peers. "I'm one of those people who bottles everything up; I get quiet, and I just sit in the corner. The dance community pushed me out of my comfort zone because people would ask me serious questions, and I'd have to think about how to answer. It's brought a lot of awareness to the foreground of not just my dance life but my work life and my love life. People are really open and communicative in the dance community. If there's something you did they didn't like, they talked about it instead of harboring resentment." That kind of communication helped her gain a lot of confidence in herself and carried over into her relationships off the dance floor—with her partner, and with her family.

Even when Alyx was a teenager, Alyx's family loved and supported her participation in dancing. "My mom is so proud of me; she brags about it to all of her friends." Her grandmother is herself a dancer—she would go dancing regularly with friends—and her grandfather plays in a blues band. "When they'd be performing at a venue that allowed underage people, they'd invite me out and watch me tear up the floor. They *love* it when I bring my friends out!"

Her favorite high school memories involve sneaking into a bar—but not to drink, to dance. "There was this long-standing blues bar in Vancouver called the Yale—it's shut down now—but Frank Sinatra used to go there. My boyfriend at the time was a regular, and he managed to get me in every Wednesday, specifically to go blues dancing. For some reason, the bouncers never looked twice—I never went to the bar to order a drink. But I used to text my mom when I was eighteen: 'OMG I got into the Yale! I get to dance tonight!' And she'd reply, 'That's so awesome!'

"I love my mother to pieces; she's an amazing woman. Last year, there was a video of me dancing that got posted on Facebook, and my mom was sharing it with everyone. At every family function we'd go to, she was like, 'Show us that video!' So, my dance life is very, very accepted in my family. They see how happy it makes me."

Not everyone is so lucky—as discussed earlier, at first glance, blues dancing can look a bit risqué. "The sensuality and intimacy of the dance was a bit of a surprise to me at first, because I started in Lindy Hop, which is a much more open position. There was one dancer—he's still in our scene, and we've become friends—who has a tango background, and when he would dance with people, he was in such close embrace. They were *right* up against each other, legs and all, and I was a little weirded out. I thought, 'That's *really* intimate. I hope he knows those people. Is he taking them out for *dinner* afterward?'" Alyx laughed.

"He still dances the exact same why, but I've noticed how my perception has changed over the years. It's easy to understand now that it's just a dance. A lot of the leads are really aware of that initial reaction from people new to the scene, so they'd ask, 'Are you okay with close embrace?' or 'Are you okay if I dip?' So it was just a matter of asking for consent. Over time I got more accustomed to the intimate nature of the dance, and I learned to love it."

In fact, she found it is the intimacy itself that makes it possible to experience that incredible dance high. "I have dances where I feel like my partner and I start as two separate beings but become a fluid body after coalescing together. You're hearing the exact same song, and even if you're not hearing it the exact same way, you're playing off each other. The energy starts building, and it starts to feel really, *really* good, and you forget that you're dancing; you're just moving and connecting and living in the moment. I always walk away from those dances being surprised. Not of myself, but just how the two of us have connected—how going into that song I had no idea that would happen, and it's utterly fantastic that it did."

Alyx got quiet and thoughtful for a moment before continuing. "You can be having the worst day of your life, but when you walk out on that floor, you forget about everything except for you and your partner and that song. I feel like dancing hasn't just taught me a physical and mental awareness—it's taught me how to be better in life, how to be healthier, how to be happier. The people who are typically involved in the blues and fusion scenes have a similar mindset—that they're here to be happy and healthy and contribute to the world in a positive way. In some other styles of dance, it feels like people are there to shut you down and make you feel small. But that's not what we do here."

I asked her what she imagined her life would be like without dance, and the ever-present smile suddenly left her face as she replied, "Without dance, I'd be a lot less happy. I think I'd still have difficulty making friends, and I'd be working in a dead-end job because of my difficulties with connecting with people and socializing. I'd be doing next to nothing because I would be in crippling pain. I wouldn't be living life to its fullest, that's for sure."

Not surprisingly, she has no plans to stop her involvement in the dance community. "I'm never going to put it down!" Alyx laughed with conviction. "Next year I'm looking at trying to enter a competition. I'm also in the process of looking to finance and start up my own traditional blues event. Event management is actually something I want to do for the long term—I love doing arts promotion and coordination. So I think that's going to be a huge piece of how dance fits into my future. I'm going to run more workshops and dance events, I'm going to try competing, and I'm going to be training a lot more."

And she'll do it whether she has social approval from her current friends or not. "I had to hit that point of frustration where I realized that if I want to do blues dancing, I can't cling to my friends to do it with me. I have to make my own friends." Thanks to her early experience with blues dancing, making new friends is no longer a problem for Alyx anyway.

I asked if she had any additional thoughts she wanted to share with readers. "Not just blues dancing, but dancing in general can open your eyes to the world and open your eyes to yourself in a way you've never experienced before. You have this ability to engage with others in a meaningful way and to get to know yourself. You build so much strength and confidence, and the way you do all of this is through music. You never would think that music would allow you to open all these doors to see yourself and *be* yourself and feel confident and secure being that person. I am ecstatic to introduce somebody to that. I want you to feel what I feel. I want you to be as happy as I feel when I dance."

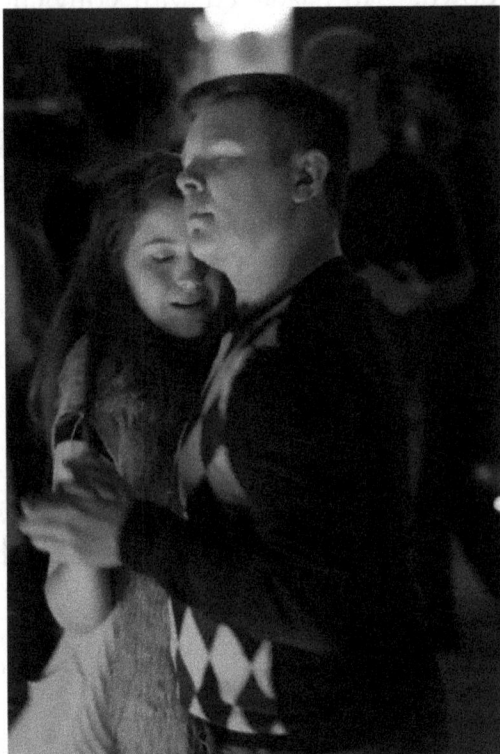

Photo by Alexey Tolstoguzov

I Learned How to Walk Again, so I Could Learn How to Dance Again

Jimmy Zamora, Sacramento, California, USA

❝You need to interview Jimmy Zamora," a fellow blues dancer told me after hearing that I was looking for stories about people who had used dance to recover from a physical limitation. "He has such an amazing story. I believe he's actually writing a book about his recovery himself." And so he is—but I'm grateful he was still open to contributing to this one. Jimmy wants to spread the word not just about how dancing can physically heal an individual but how it has the potential to heal the planet.

Jimmy got involved in social dancing after his life took a severe turn—but not the physical one that derailed his life. That came later. He first went through a divorce and a career change—after twelve years of marriage and eighteen years working for newspapers, he transitioned to being a single parent working in politics. He met a new woman whom he liked, who happened to be a dancer. She practiced West Coast swing dancing, but she knew Jimmy was more of a blues music kind of guy. She encouraged him to try blues dancing, and he did. He attended a blues fusion dance event in March 2011 and thoroughly loved it.

"One of the things that struck me about it is that I'm a talker and a writer—words just pour out of me; you squeeze me, and they come out—and dance is a social encounter that I couldn't talk my way through. Dance is a different language. That was a complete challenge for me, but a beautiful one. I'm learning this whole new way to communicate, and it came at a point in life when I needed an emotional reset button."

Jimmy's physical reset button came next. Only a month after attending his first blues dance event, he woke up one morning feeling completely numb on the left side of his body. By the end of the day, it had started to spread, so he checked into the emergency room. He thought he might be having a stroke; the doctor assured him it was not a stroke, although he didn't know what it was. Jimmy was told to go home that night, and if it was still bothering him when he woke up, to come back to the hospital the next day. It would more than bother him. The next morning, he woke up and couldn't walk. The condition had spread to both his legs.

"It wasn't that I was paralyzed. I could still wiggle my toes and lift my legs, but I'd lost effective control of my muscles. Something zapped through me. I woke up in the morning, my dog wanted to go to the bathroom, I needed to feed my daughter breakfast, and I can't walk. So I'm dragging myself and pushing on walls trying to balance myself. Finally, I was able to get someone to pick up my daughter, and I got a ride to the hospital. I didn't come back home after that for a month."

It turned out to be a condition called transverse myelitis—a neurological condition related to inflammation of the spinal cord, whose symptoms overlap a lot with multiple sclerosis symptoms. Some patients are symptom-free six months later; others show signs of improvement up to two years later, and others may never show signs of recovery. "I was terrified that first morning. I didn't know how serious it was."

Jimmy immediately entered spinal rehab and remained there for three weeks. "They essentially taught me how to walk again." A characteristic of Jimmy's ailment is that his muscles still function properly, but he can lose all muscle memory. "We all learn to walk as toddlers but to have to learn how to do it again forty years later is crazy—it's really easy to overthink. With this condition, my feet were almost numb, so it was hard to feel the floor. It's scary. You've got to learn to trust."

They sent him home with a wheelchair, but he was determined to learn how to walk again, so he could learn how to dance again. "Even when I was in a wheelchair in rehab, I would lean back and put my feet in the air and move them to the beat of music." He used a walker before transitioning to crutches and then later a cane.

"I went to a lot of physical therapy, and dance classes are the best physical therapy—blues is one of the best forms of physical therapy." Even though it was not long before he stopped using his walker to walk, he used it to teach himself how to dance. He set up two walkers and stood in the middle of them, rocking back and forth between them. He still had poor balance, but he felt safe that he'd have something to grab on to. "It was like a game; I'd spread the circle a little further apart and just rock my feet back and forth and begin to incorporate slides."

Eventually, he worked up enough coordination and courage to attend a blues dance. He wasn't sure he'd be able to dance with a partner yet, but at one point a man who was bigger than him offered. "Try it. Dance with me." As those who are new to blues dancing are likely beginning to learn through these stories, it is not uncommon for a male to dance with a male or a female to dance with another female. What is uncommon is to have to do so out of necessity.

"He could hold me up, so I danced with him like four times that night. I wanted to cry. I was like, 'God, I can actually dance again!' I mean, I was terrible at it, but it became a passion of mine." By late 2012, Jimmy started feeling really comfortable with partner dancing again. "It took a year or so of practice before then, where I wasn't really progressing, but I was doing it because I loved it and I had to do it. I felt it deep inside—I couldn't live with myself if I didn't dance."

Blues dancing was the perfect introduction back into the dance world for Jimmy.
"I always liked the music and the connection, and I realized that I could do it because you can dance small with blues. I could dance small and still give someone a good experience. Having a medical challenge to overcome forced me to become a different kind of dancer than I would have been otherwise. I've learned to be a better listener through dancing. I earned a living

by being a talker, but everyone communicates different in dance. With some people, you have to learn how to hear them. Since I was the guy who had the fewest moves, by keeping it open, I was saying to the other person, 'What do you want to do? This is your opportunity to embellish, to design, to communicate with me.'"

As Jimmy said, there's no such thing as a bad dance anyway. "A dance is still a dance even if it's not the best dance. Even if it's some beginner who steps on your toes, whose arms turn into spaghetti, she still gave you a dance. The music played, and you were on the dance floor with a wonderful human being. The other night, someone stepped on my toes—someone else's follow, and wearing a heel. She apologized to me later in the night, and I said, 'My feet are already numb, so if you're going to step on someone's feet, it may as well be mine.'"

Gradually, however, Jimmy has been able to gain some sensitivity back in his feet by incorporating physical therapy into every moment of his life. "I used to walk my dog barefoot around the block because it increased the sensitivity in my feet; it helped wake up nerve endings. When I brush my teeth, I practice standing on one leg, or I cook while on one leg. I have a workstation at my job where the desk can be raised, so I can stand, and I'll work while standing on one foot."

While he was in recovery, Jimmy didn't go back to work for several months. "I burned up all my sick time and most of my vacation time. I came really close

to filing for permanent disability. I definitely qualified."
He did go back to working on political campaigns
eventually, however, and he noticed a correlation
between yeses in dance and those given through voting.
"One of the things I realized is nobody ever wins an
election by converting 'no' votes to yeses; you win by
finding more votes that are 'yes' from the start."
Therefore, he doesn't get hung up on the people who
don't enjoy his dance style—he instead focuses on the
yeses. "I work to my fans." He laughed.

No matter what, he's always felt welcomed by
the blues fusion community. "Most of the people in my
life before dance were writers. They understood my
humor, the speed at which my brain was moving, et
cetera. But the people I've met through dance…the way
they've embraced me—it's such a beautiful thing. After
all those years of being a journalist and PR person, being
really well-known in media—these dancers didn't know
me at all. I didn't exist on any of those planes for them.
I'm just a dude who's asking them to dance."

Even though Jimmy has "a ton of friends," his
physical condition can still leave him feeling lonely.
"When you first wake up in the morning, and your
balance is off, and you need the support of the wall, it's
a lonely and scary thing. So the fact that people still
want to dance with me—that's the pot of gold at the
end of the rainbow. It's a powerful form of emotional
validation that this journey was worth it."

Physical contact played a big role in Jimmy's
health—even outside of the role it played in his physical

recovery. "The intimacy of blues is backed up by the culture. Connection with others has been fundamentally healing to me, because a blues dance is kind of a hug. Hugs heal. Even before I got sick, it was good for me. Coming out of a divorce, there were levels of intimacy I was having trouble with. But from the blues dance culture, I've learned that you can have a pretty intense romance within a three-minute song. That was fulfilling something for me before I got sick, and then after I got sick, I appreciated it in a totally profound new way. I recognized it was really nourishing for me—I'd come back home after a dance, and I'd just feel this *high*."

That emotional high carried over in his workday as well. "I'm so much better, so much happier at work, the day after a night out dancing. I've never had a bad night of dancing. I work in a profession that is extremely energy draining. I'll leave work wearing a suit and tie, coming from a crazy political thing, and one little voice in me is saying, 'You're totally wiped—just go home and relax,' and the other voice says, 'You've never regretted dancing. Ever. Just go and do it for an hour.' But 99.9 percent of the time, I end up staying until it ends.

"A dance is more than a dance. It's an emotional thing; I'm in a space where it's safe for me to be vulnerable. In the political arena, you can't actually be vulnerable unless it's in a way that makes you appear stronger. But with blues, I can just be me—it's okay. I can be vulnerable there. As soon as I walk into a dance, my stress level goes down. I go in there and slide my tie off, and I'm home."

I asked Jimmy if he believes dancing could change the world, and he related how it could begin to do so by altering the personalities of some of the worst people he crossed paths with in the political world.

"I know a lot of jerks in the world, but I don't know many on the dance floor at all. I think if more people danced, it would decrease the percentage of people that are jerks. Dance teaches good lessons as far as socialization. All women have stories about men who said or did something that made them feel very uncomfortable. That can happen sometimes on the dance floor, but it happens a lot less, because it's a culture of consent. You have to ask, and you have to be nice, or no one's going to want to dance with you. The market speaks."

As far as I could tell, Jimmy had no problem finding his own following—and he is more than ready to wave the blues banner.

"I'd like to have my last dance be on my last day of life, when I'm over one hundred. As long as someone's willing to dance with me, I'll dance. And that person who's willing to dance with me can be me."

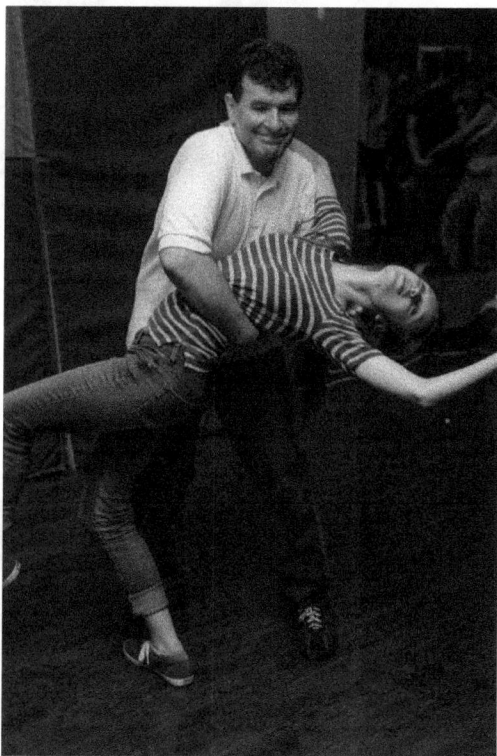

Photo by Shane Meyers/Speakeasy Photos

III
MIND

The mind can make or break your well-being. It can take you to deep, daunting places—memories of the past as much as fears about the future. What dancing has done for so many people is offer something to hold on to in the midst of mental crisis.

Many interviewees said something along these lines: "If I can just get through X number of days, the next day, I get to go dancing." What happens on the dance floor is a landmark transition to distract us—or temporarily relieve us—from the thoughts that normally occupy our minds. If those aren't often happy thoughts, life can seem dark and unforgiving.

The following stories provide evidence that the mind doesn't have to stay in whatever state it's currently in. For some contributors to this section, even if it takes everything they have to get out bed or to leave the house, when they walk onto the dance floor, the effort becomes worth it. That temporary fix may even become permanent. These six individuals have used dancing as a starting point to shift their minds to healthier states.

Comfortable in My Own Skin

Laura K., Milan, Italy

❝Blues as a dance is totally new in Italy. We don't have a blues scene yet, but I'm helping to start one in Milan." Laura is a woman of initiative. She wasn't always so courageous, however. Her journey to being the confident, self-expressive woman that she is began on the blues dance floor.

It was only a couple of years ago that an international dance teacher came to Genoa, Italy, to teach a mixed workshop—a collection of Lindy Hop and balboa with a blues taster. Laura liked the blues class right away, but it was only a minor portion of the event, and there was no opportunity to dance it at the social that night.

Later, however, leaders in the European blues dance scene, Vicci Moore and Adamo Ciarallo, came from London to teach a workshop. Not only was this workshop exclusively on blues but so was the evening social—the teachers brought along six or seven people from their London classes to attend the dance that night. This made all the difference. "We actually had a chance to watch and dance with people who had been blues dancing for a couple of years. It was different than just seeing the teachers dance, because your mind labels them 'teachers,' and you start to think, 'I won't be able to dance like them, so I'm not even going to try.' But these other people were people like us—not teachers—

so dancing with them is what made it click for us," Laura explained. "As a beginner, if the teacher just shows you a couple of moves, and that's all you get to practice, you will eventually get bored. But if you dance with someone else who knows more moves, and he or she shows you that you can be creative beyond the moves you learned in class, it's a very different experience. So I think that was the turning point."

The turning point Laura spoke of was finding a style of dance—and a community—where she could feel comfortable in her own skin. "Dancing is something I always liked doing as a child. But I've never been a thin girl; I've always been quite chubby. When I was a kid, I wanted to go to ballet classes, but my father told me, 'You're not fit for that kind of thing,' and he wouldn't bring me to ballet. For years, I buried my desire to dance and the ache that I felt." It wasn't until Laura reached college that she started exploring the idea of dancing again. She began solo dancing at parties; she had the awareness that she was naturally able to move to the beat and subtleties of the music, but she continued to feel that she wasn't elegant or "sexy" enough to dance where others could see her. "I loved dancing, but I did it in the corner. I didn't dance with the rest of the party."

By the time she was in her midthirties, she had found the courage to experiment with partner dancing. "I started by taking Italian folk dancing—which was more a cultural activity than it was dancing—before trying tango for a couple of years. I was a control freak, so I thought maybe if I learned to follow and had to dance 90 percent of the time backward, then that might help balance my control issue." Laura laughed in spite of herself, recalling the person she'd been not long ago. "So going to tango was half like going to therapy, half dancing."

Lindy Hop came next. "Six or seven years ago I was very involved with photography, and I had the chance to take photographs at burlesque shows. At one point during a show, there were these people dancing Lindy Hop. I didn't know what it was, but I thought they looked like they were having the time of their lives, so I wanted to try it. I tried to find a place to dance it, but I couldn't find one, so I gave up. Then three years ago I met a friend of mine in the subway, and I asked her where she was going and she said, 'I'm going to a boogie-woogie class.' I said, 'Okay! I'm going too!'"

Laura's immediate reaction was that the community welcomed her, even when she came alone and did not know anyone there. She liked the people and the environment, but after a while she found that the dance only allowed her to convey a very specific and limited set of emotions while being "too jumpy." She also found it difficult to quell the voice in her head saying, "You're not looking good enough with this." She knew she was able to pick up moves very easily, but she still thought she didn't look "right" on the outside. In addition, her "control issues" were still in effect—she didn't like the lack of freedom to style, or occasionally lead, her own moves.

"With Lindy Hop, you can add your personal interpretation to the dance, but it's very technical. I'm not saying blues is not technical—I get mad when someone says that. Blues is just as technical as Lindy Hop, but it's more about having the right posture or moving the right way not to injure yourself."

When she found blues, she found the perfect balance. "In blues, you can have classes where they teach you variations, but they encourage you to do it in your own way. And that really frees you. It's easier to compromise with your partner. I could still be in the role of the follow, but I have the option of breaking away and doing something I hear in the music that my lead does not. My feet could be doing one thing with my partner, while my upper body does something else. It's like having a conversation with my partner without shouting at him; if he doesn't want to have a conversation with the music, I can have my own."

Laura discovered that she could also dance by herself—with the rest of the party this time—and have that be perfectly all right. Sometimes even preferable. "Maybe I don't feel like inviting someone else to dance; maybe I really like the song, and I don't want it to be affected by someone else's interpretation of it. I just want to dance to it the way I feel it and the way I hear it. The only relationship I want to have in that moment is with the music."

Being able to dance alone in public was a big step for Laura. "I always used to check if someone was looking at me, but I don't do that anymore. I don't care what they're thinking. I don't care, and at the same time I know I don't look so bad. Maybe I'm not the best dancer in the world—for sure I'm not the best dancer in the world—but I look like someone that is having fun, and looking at someone that is having fun is always something nice."

Laura found that the blues scene lacked the competitiveness that she'd found in other dance forms, and wherever she went, the community continued to amaze her with its openness. "I've been to two blues dance events in London, one in Barcelona, and one in Tel Aviv. I've met people from the United States, from northern Europe, Eastern Europe, from wherever, and what I find defines a blues dancer is acceptance. Wherever I go, I instantly feel this welcoming feeling. We would do things in community—we'd go to classes, then have a picnic together, then go back to the venue for the dance. I'd be in the ladies' room exchanging makeup with women I've never met—women saying, 'I can do your hair if you want!'"

Laura recognized, however, her tendency to get too attached to people with whom she shared a connection. Especially in a culture where the people you meet are often not from your own country, the likelihood of never seeing each other again is real. That was a hard lesson for Laura to learn at first. "It's always been difficult for me to get close to someone else. So when I find somebody interesting, and we establish a connection, it is very hard for me to let go. I've felt like, 'Okay, so now I found you, and you made me laugh, and I find you interesting, so let's stick together!'" Laura laughed and held her arms to her chest in a mock embrace.

"This wasn't okay. So this is what I learned when I started dancing blues—you can have this lump in your throat and be very touched and deeply moved by your dance partner, and then say thank you and accept that you might not see each other again. You have to be happy for what you had instead of being sad because you'll never have that again."

At the same time, however, Laura recognizes that there can be a form of healthy attachment. She frequently travels in order to partake in the dance at a higher level, so often her path *will* cross with those she thought she'd never see again. "If I want to dance blues, I have to travel. This is one of the reasons my friend and I decided to start this social in Milan—we were spending a lot of money traveling around Europe just to dance blues." Laura admits that even when her local scene has grown, however, she will likely still travel for dance. "I've met so many people through attending festivals. This may sound strong, but I really feel that some of them are my family at this point. My scattered-around-Europe family, but still my family."

Another valuable lesson Laura acquired through dancing is how to connect with others on a non-cerebral level. "I've never been the kind of girl who can go to a party and flirt with someone and make out. All of my relationships and sexual experiences in college were the outcome of a very long and deep intellectual conversation where you get to know me, I get to know you, we say very interesting or funny or brilliant things, and *then* we make out. I didn't trust the way I communicated with my body, so I'd always felt that the only way for me to be attractive is by showing you my brain, so I never even tried another way, I didn't know how to do it.

"Then I found blues, and I learned how to communicate with the way I move my hips, or the way I lay my hand on someone's shoulder, and I saw how things started to change. I could go to socials and dance with someone, and after a couple of dances and chats we could eventually kiss, even though we might not see each other again. I discovered that it's okay, that I can do that. This is something that girls know how to do when they're fifteen, and I've learned it now at forty-two, so it's a bit late but not too late."

It's hard to imagine Laura ever took herself so seriously. The version of her that I know now is one that freely expresses joy and wears an ever-present smile. Her hair color is different every time a photo of her crosses my social media feed—most often a shade of pink. Her mannerisms are feminine, confident, and friendly. That's not the way her friends always perceived her, though. "One of my friends used to tell me that I wasn't able to have a conversation that wasn't serious." Laura grinned with a look of guilt that demonstrated there was an element of truth to that. "Maybe now I'm more able to have a silly or emotional chat with someone else without getting brainy."

Laura is definitely aware of her increase in confidence. She has recently even begun her own social dance event with a friend in Milan. Each social opens with a beginner blues class, which took a lot of courage for her to decide to teach with her friend. "We questioned if we could handle the responsibility. We like to think of ourselves as tools; we show people the tip of the iceberg, and then if they want to continue with the dance, they can go to workshops or festivals and learn from regular teachers."

Nevertheless, she has to work through fear every time the class comes around.

"I'm scared to death every night we do this. Maybe no one will show up, or maybe we'll screw up during the class, or maybe people won't dance. But when people come, and they are involved in the class, and they stay and dance all night, I get such a burst of energy. I've never felt that before. I wouldn't have been able to do that one year ago. It takes some confidence in yourself to say, 'Okay, I'm able to do that; I'm able to talk to venues and put together classes to teach and be the point of reference for these people.' But I've learned that I can do it. I can show people what blues dancing is and try to make them love it"—Laura paused before adding with a playful smile—"even though it won't be as much as I do."

Laura expressed fear when she talked about teaching, but she also expressed pride.

"It was really powerful the first time I taught at our social in Milan. I didn't know I could show people how to groove and to move—how to explain it. At some point we were teaching them a turn, and I looked around the room, and everybody was doing it! I was like, 'Ahh! They are so good!' It was like having children and teaching them how to tie their shoes or something; you're so proud. But not proud of me—I didn't feel like *I* did this; I was like *they're* doing this. And I didn't even know them—I was proud of strangers." Laura's face took on a look of amazement, once again not of herself but of the magic that is possible on the dance floor.

Like most people who reach this level of involvement with the dance community, Laura cannot imagine her future without dance playing an integral role.

She still maintains a shadow of her former life, being employed at a digital marketing company. She is specialized in the fashion and luxury industries, and whereas many women dream about getting paid to browse shoes and handbags, Laura wants to do something else with her life. "Ideally, I would like to quit my job and make my life all about dancing, but I don't suppose that's realistic." Her free time, however, is almost entirely about dancing.

"Outside of work, I am social dancing, rehearsing dancing, putting together playlists for dancing, or teaching people to dance. And I do it all mostly for free. I'm not complaining, though; I would do it again and again."

When I asked what her biggest challenge was regarding teaching blues dancing, her answer came as a surprise. It wasn't worrying about what other people thought about how she looked. Rather, it was helping others overcome body image issues that come with their ideas of dancing a "sexy dance."

"With people who don't know anything about blues dancing, it's easier. However, with Lindy Hoppers or people who have had some small experience with blues dancing who think, 'I'm not fit for blues dancing because I'm not sexy,' or, 'I don't want to grind myself with another person's body,' I have to explain to them that it's not like that. Sometimes the best dances I have are silly ones where we laugh the whole time; we're not trying to be sexy at all—we're just having fun. Sexy is not something that comes before blues; it is something that comes *after* blues, because you become confident in the way you dance, and then you become sexy, because you're confident. It's not something you need to have before you start dancing. You don't have to be sexy to be a good blues dancer. But you might *become* a very sexy person if you dance blues."

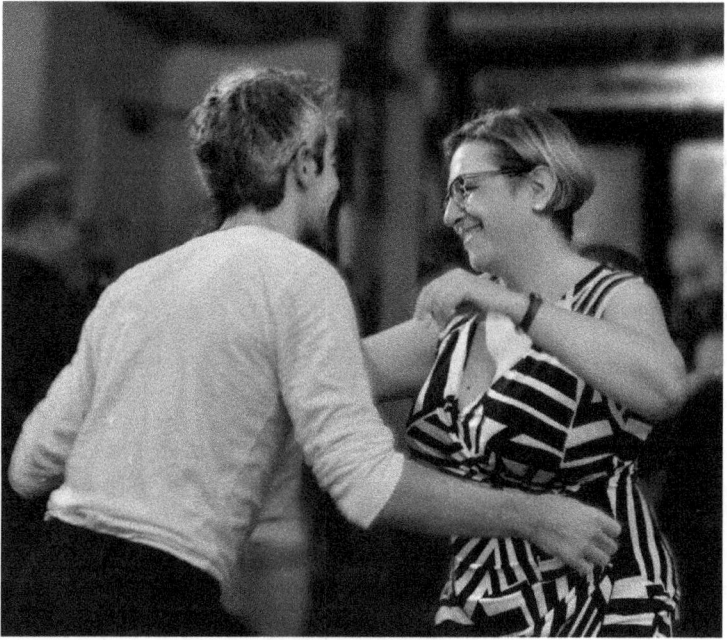

Photo by Fabio Bortot

Dancing out of Darkness

Clara Pochettino, London, England

I first met Clara while attending a blues dance class in London. We were paired up to do an exercise in which the follow was blindfolded. Clara was my lead; I had to trust her to guide me around the room without walking me into an object or another couple. What I recalled most almost a year later was that Clara was a great guide; her indications were subtle yet clear, and her words were enthusiastic and encouraging. Her natural exuberance effortlessly compensated for my quiet character.

I was delighted, therefore, when she approached me weeks later after I'd made an announcement that I was seeking stories of transformation for this book. I knew she wouldn't have any problem opening up; mostly I would just need to listen and allow her story to come through naturally. Her excitement was contagious as she declared, "Blues dancing changed my life." I wouldn't find out *how* it changed her life until several months later, however, when I returned to London and we sat down in a quiet corner of a posh hotel lobby. Hanging above Clara's head was a black-and-white portrait of Audrey Hepburn. As she was bundled in a long black coat and wearing a furry, shiny black hat atop her platinum-blond hair, Clara's own elegance and beauty complemented that of the portrait's subject. I felt like I was interviewing a movie star.

"I dressed up for the interview, in case you wanted to take my picture." Clara tilted her head toward her shoulder and flashed a glowing smile. "Just kidding, just kidding." I suspected that Clara would love to lead a trail of paparazzi, all joking aside.

Our interview began. Reminiscent of our initial encounter, she was a natural leader, requiring very little prompting for her story to pour out. I began as I did most interviews for this book: I asked how she first discovered blues dancing.

"A couple of years ago I was into this new plan of trying things out. There was no dance in my life, so I decided to explore it. So, when a friend invited me to try this blues dance that nobody knew about in London—it was quite a new scene—I decided to give it a go, and after the first lesson, I understood that the lag from when you begin to when you start enjoying it is ten minutes, and I said sure, straight away, this is my dance!" Clara's face lit up as she recalled the moment.

Clara was from Italy, and I wasn't sure if blues music had much of a presence there. I asked her if she was already familiar with the music, or if her first introduction to it was on the dance floor.

"I did hear blues music before, without knowing it was blues. The first record I ever bought was blues music, when I was probably seven or eight years old, and I remember listening to it continuously. That was at my dad's place, and then we lost the record—it was on gramophone. I always liked blues music; I've always felt a strong connection to it. And now, because I've been living in London for ten years, I'm able to understand the words of the songs as well. Previously, the connection to the music had always been to the rhythm and the feel, not really to the words. I couldn't understand a thing! So now, there is another interesting angle to the music for me to appreciate."

Although my immediate impression of Clara was that she was a confident and joyful woman, she revealed that at the time she began blues dancing, she was a very different person. "I liked the music, I liked the rhythm, but since I'd never danced before, I didn't have any technique. In the beginning, I was all in my head, wondering, 'Am I doing this right?' I also had a real problem allowing other people into my space, so for me, physical contact with another person, especially with a man, was difficult for me.

"So at the end of the hour, I was sweating, not only from the exercise but also from the emotional pressure. I couldn't take any more. I had to stop. It's shifted now; now I can't stop—you have to drag me away from the dance floor! I could dance with a camel, if I found the willingness. So it has changed—gradually but constantly—and now I've discovered a part of myself that I'd cut myself off from for many years."

Clara's excitement gave way to a deep moment of reflection. Her face fell into a peaceful state, and she paused briefly before continuing,

"My life has changed so deeply. I'd had a series of experiences that led me into maybe twenty months of depression. I didn't go out from my house after work.

Work was enough for me—I couldn't take anymore. And even going to work sometimes was really, really hard. It left me exhausted, and I didn't have any space for social interaction—especially nothing as challenging as getting physically close to someone. Something shifted before I started dancing, of course—I was already open enough to go to a dance class on my own—but dancing provided a safe space for me to practice what I'd been talking about with my therapist. I could see what my dynamic with the outside world was, and with men specifically. How was I reacting to the presence of a man in my space? I slowly learned to let go of my anxiety."

Her anxiety wasn't the only thing Clara let go of as a result of dance. "Interestingly enough, when I started dancing, I was a smoker! I always had been for twenty or more years, but then because of dancing, it became important for me to have very nice breath, so I gave up smoking." Clara laughed in awe of herself. "I mean, that was really something unachievable, as silly as it is, but for me to be so close to someone, I had to not smell bad. I also understood that my need to smoke was a cover over insecurity. I practiced getting over my insecurity by asking people to dance with me. When I broke down the wall by asking strangers to dance with me, I took the first major step in the recovery from my previous life. It felt so scary, and yet it was the most courageous thing that I've ever done."

Clara attested that having music and dance in her life at least once a week felt like a regular visit to a therapist. "Dancing became a constant and very important appointment not to miss. The most important appointment in my life." And the rewards from that one appointment were plentiful. "I'm not very good technically, but the shift in my soul has been huge. Huge emotionally and physically. I've learned to accept my body, to accept that someone else is looking at me while I dance. All those things were not in my previous life at all.

"Blues dancing is something I will always be grateful for. I'm incredibly grateful for the people I've met who immediately helped me feel peace. They didn't set targets or make comparisons. It's not a competitive environment; it's very welcoming. I remember my teacher telling us at the very beginning, 'Don't worry about doing it right. You need to find your own voice. You need to find your own blues.' For me, that meant even more than learning how to technically move. I had to find how *Clara* feels the moves, how *Clara* feels this music. No one had ever said anything like that to me before, and it's not easy to find that in any other kind of dance. With blues, even if it's not technically perfect, spontaneity and enthusiasm can make up for what's lacking."

Clara's earlier statement that blues dancing had changed her life was strong. I wanted to know what other layers of transformation had not yet been uncovered, so I asked how dancing had carried over into other areas of her life.

Clara continued thoughtfully, "You know, I've started looking at my life as a dance, my job as a dance. I'm an accountant, and I remember last year I was going around the office trying a new walk or the fish tail in front of the copy machine, and that raised more than one eyebrow." She chuckled at the memory. "I was trying to convince them how accounting is actually like a dance, because I'd just come from a workshop where we were doing connection exercises. Without touching, the follow had to mirror exactly the moves of the lead. So, for me, that brought this idea that every action has a reaction and actually everything is in balance, like in my balance sheet. There are these debits and credits, and everything mirrors everything else.

"I also learned from dance how to ask for what I want. For me, that was a major handicap. I asked people to dance with me, and I found out that it wasn't that tough. I mean, it was *really* tough, but it was over quickly. You can ask, they can say no, and sometimes it's personal, but most of the time it's not. It's just because people are tired, or they were going for a break, or they promised themselves to someone else. That gave me a completely different perspective about other areas of my life—how to ask for a promotion or a pay raise, how to ask my flatmates for what I needed in the house, how to ask my parents for what I needed in my life. And not just how to communicate my needs but mostly how to accept their answer, understanding that it wasn't always about me. If it was a refusal, that was okay.

"I remember receiving feedback from a dance partner once when he told me that I was, for him, one of the easiest follows to dance with. I think that for one week I was in heaven, in pure joy. I felt like, more than my quality as a follow, it was validation as a human being. It was an acceptance of Clara as a person; it means that I'm able to listen, it means that I'm able to follow, to use signals. It was probably so meaningful because for me it was so hard in the beginning to let go and relax. When that compliment came along, nothing has ever meant so much.

"There are times, however, when I have an unenjoyable experience during a dance. Learning that I can put up with a little bit of discomfort for a few minutes has been therapeutic. In the past, I would enter into a social relationship or be in a social environment and think, 'I don't know when this ends,' and that gave me a lot of anxiety. Instead, if I know that it's for the length of a song, then that makes me feel better. So even if I'm not totally comfortable in a situation, I can teach myself to breathe, relax, and recently even to enjoy, as long as they don't hurt me.

"That has been a valuable lesson to learn how to say stop, to move away from a space where I'm not comfortable. Coming from a history of trauma, in the past I would either run away without saying anything, or I would just not put myself in a social position in the first place, preventing me from having an experience. It could be a good experience or a bad experience, but who knows?

"So even if I had an uncomfortable experience, I kept going back. Having a core group of people who are always there made it easier for me, so if I have a bad dance, then I can go ask one of my trusted leads, 'Can I dance with you? I need to breathe and refocus, because for the moment I'm all over the place.' And everything is good again, and I remember why I love dancing."

Her relationship with the music has deepened as well. "The music honestly does the majority of the work. Blues music is soothing on a level that nothing else is for me. It calms me; it makes me feel peace. I think it's the longing…this feeling of sadness that I can relate to on some level. I really feel like it's talking to me, to my soul.

"I've even started playing the harmonica. Listening to blues songs, the harmonica is a really important part, and I like the sound of it. So at the beginning of last year I contacted a teacher, and I took some private lessons. Now I'm a not-very-good harmonica player." Clara laughed. "Music didn't exist in my life before; nobody in my family plays an instrument. In Italy…I know that you guys think that we are all poets and singers, but we're not."

Clara paused long enough for me to divulge that, in fact, I could tell already that she *was* a poet. Her words flowed so readily and artfully that I found myself captivated by her story. I wanted to know more. I asked her to tell me about her relationship with her family. Did they support her dancing?

"Well, my family is difficult by default, so I'm not too worried about what they think of my dancing. They didn't really manifest any enthusiasm. They question the fact that I'm a bit old to start a new life. They wonder why don't I instead do something useful for my job, like learn a new skill that I can actually use in my field. Well, because it's boring." Clara raised her hand as if brushing the thought aside. "I want to do something joyful!"

In fact, dancing has influenced all of her relationships—not just with her family.

"It opened a totally new set of friendships and dynamics. I need authentic people in my life, I need the relationship to be sincere. A person won't stay in my world if we don't exchange something pure. Especially after the depression, this became a requirement.

"Dancing is a wonderful way to connect meaningfully with another person. If I dance with you, I kind of know you in a very intimate way. I understand from the way that we dance together if a person is curious, if he's fearful, if he likes to stick to what he knows or if he's adventurous, if he stays in the moment, and if he sees who he's dancing with. Does he know that it's Clara? Is he listening to my needs or to my level of dancing? I find that this kind of knowledge is something so precious. It can never be grasped from a regular conversation with a partner or any other way of meeting people that I have experienced before."

I asked Clara if there was a particular moment or dance that stood out for her as extra meaningful. As with all her answers, she entered into another heartfelt silique that really made me feel she should be a writer herself—or a storyteller. She gazed upward introspectively, and answered,

"Yes, dancing in the street in Madrid. I was dancing with a guy who was there at the dance festival I was attending. He was a very, *very* cute guy. And I was thinking, 'Clara, this is like a dream come true. You are dancing, swinging in the air with this lovely man in a lovely place.' It's something that if I had thought about it a couple months before, it would not even have seemed possible. It wasn't in my reality. And now, I'm able to dance with no shame. I'm not thinking about myself, my body, or how I look. I'm just feeling. I'm just feeling the connection, and I'm enjoying this very moment."

"How do you see dance fitting into your future?" I asked.

Clara smiled with a dreamy expression and replied, "I see dance very present in my future. Very much so. I want to dance forever. I want to live a life that allows me to dance regularly and to travel to festivals. I need to make more money. Before when I was depressed, I could live on what I am making, but now I have lots of things to do, places to be, I need to be everywhere!"

I relished watching Clara come alive with the possibilities.

"And I need to buy nice dresses and comfortable shoes. Dancing changed the way that I shop for clothes.

Now I don't buy a dress if I don't think I can dance in it."

Clara's vision for the future turned to romantic relationships, and she grew silent for a few moments before continuing. "I think that if I could dance every day, even two minutes, that a potential relationship could have a chance. Because I understand that there is a way to connect—with myself and with another person. I know that whatever happens, I can go back to that. So I need to find a dancing partner, someone who agrees to be dragged to dance lessons." She laughed at the predicament her future partner might encounter.

In the meantime, Clara's life is robust with positive relationships and connections—many of which she's taking the lead on forming.

"I make it a point to invite one or two new dancers to dance every night. I can see them standing close to the wall, and I've been there—I know how hard it is to go and ask someone to dance. I make it my rule to always leave them with a compliment, always something encouraging. Even if it seems there's nothing to say because it was really bad, I can say, 'I can see you have potential. Why don't you come to classes?' I want to give back a little bit of the confidence that I took from this community, because it gave me a new life. I haven't been to that dark place in ages...months!"

I could have listened to Clara speak for hours, but our time together was drawing to a close. I asked her if she had any final thoughts she wanted to share about what she'd learned about herself through dancing.

"The other day I danced with a guy, and I couldn't believe he asked me to dance again. I thought, 'Are you nuts? We almost killed each other, didn't we?'" Clara laughed. "So apparently for him it wasn't the same experience that it was for me." Clara turned her head with a sly smile. "I said no. I don't usually say no. That's also something that I'm questioning in my life: why do I never say no? My manager puts something on my desk, and I can't say no, can I? It never occurred to me that I could say that! Why? Because I'm grateful, I'm so pleased that I have the opportunity for this job, because it's such an honor, and because I'm not good at doing anything else, so thank you. Dancing has given me a safe place, like a gym where I can train my muscles, to say yes, to say no, to notice my reactions, how I feel.

"I also have the freedom of changing some behaviors. Where else in society do I have this opportunity to practice, in a safe way? I find it easier to talk to people about my needs now. I went to my manager, and I said, 'You know what—I do a good job. I think I deserve a pay raise.' I would never have done that before in my life. And I got it! If I didn't ask, they certainly weren't coming to me at all. So I did ask. And it was difficult, but not as difficult as I thought it would be. And I think it's because I practice staying in a slightly difficult situation for three minutes sometimes. In another space, but those are transferable skills to have and use in my life. I'm using what I've learned. I'm using it at work; I'm using it with my family. I'm dancing through life. And I find it amazing.

"And there's one more thing. Last year the local dance teachers here in London gave us the opportunity to perform for Christmas. They gave us the space to offer up a performance. They let us decide what we wanted to do, just come up with something exciting. So I decided to do a solo. Before, dancing with a partner was really challenging for me, but then it became very comfortable, and instead it was really challenging when I was left alone—but I'm finding my own voice.

"Actually, someone took a picture of me during my solo performance. I'm going to show you this picture because you know, words are lovely, but images reveal so much more. Look. I have problems even recognizing myself. See that? Am I not happy? I was so incredibly happy."

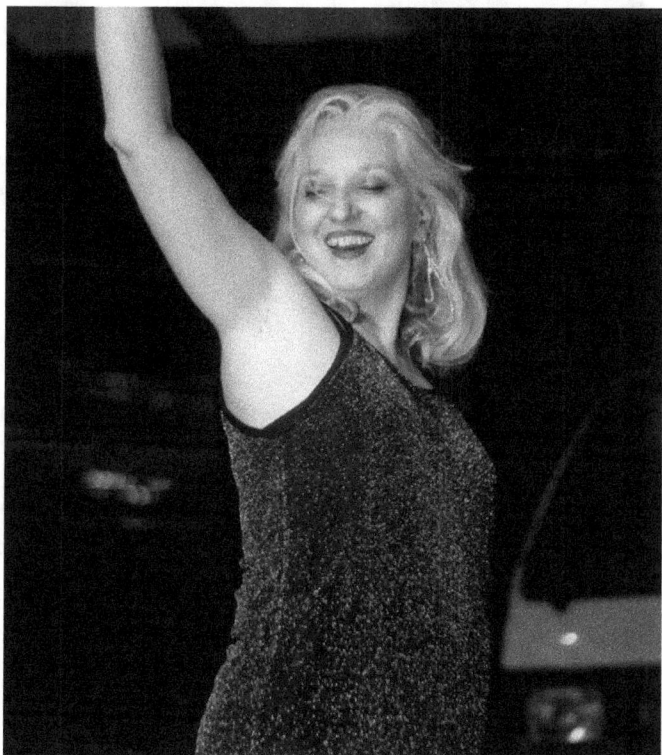

Photo by Fredrik Lindbom

Replacing Military Memories with Magical Moments

Ryan Limbaugh, Portland, Oregon, USA

I had seen Ryan at dances several times over the years, as we both reside in Portland, Oregon. However, we officially became acquainted over me screaming in terror. We were volunteering to help the organizers of an upcoming Blues Recess event prepare the build materials for the floating dance floor—among other artistic endeavors. The materials had not been used since last year's event and instead lay collecting dust and other debris alongside a Southeast Portland home—creating the perfect conditions for a colony of mice.

Upon lifting one particular log, I released the beasts. What appeared to be nearly one hundred baby mice scattered in every direction—a few across my feet. Other volunteers in the general vicinity came over to assess the source of my outcry, one of whom was Ryan. However, his reaction was distinctly different than mine. "Oh, they're so cute!" Despite his ambivalence to what had left me utterly squeamish, Ryan was compassionate. He offered to take over the project at hand, and my lungs—and heart—remain grateful to this day.

What occurred out of this uncomfortable encounter, however, was the opportunity to sit down with Ryan and uncover the layers of emotional trauma from which he'd been able to find relief through dancing.

Ryan served in the military for three years, half of which was spent overseas in Iraq and Kuwait. His life had significant challenges even before then. "My parents divorced when I was twelve. I had a lot of support from each of them individually, but not a whole lot of open-mindedness. I was out of the house by fifteen, living with friends. After high school, the only options I was aware of were to go to college or go to the military. I'd been a terrible student, barely earning my high school degree, so I knew school was not for me. I had an uncle and a friend in the military, so going to the military seemed like the obvious choice."

A week after receiving his high school diploma, Ryan was sent to Fort Benning in Georgia. He excelled there and made corporal rank E4 really quickly. What came after that, Ryan seemed averse to wanting to share, and I did not press the issue. His path to healing was the subject at hand, and in that, blues dancing played an integral part.

"I discovered blues dancing about a year after I got out of the military. It was ten years ago now. I had a friend who told me, 'You *have* to come blues dancing.' I gave her all these excuses as to why I couldn't, and she just put her finger on my mouth and said, 'Shhh!'

"So, I finally went with her to a dance. I hadn't done any partner dancing at all before that, and I left there basically in love with it. I continued to go to a lot of beginner lessons after that and just drank it in."

Unexpectedly, that decision to go dancing led to Ryan reestablishing purpose in his life. "After I returned from the military, I had a lot of drive and maturity, but I had no direction. I wasn't really invested in anything; I was just paying the bills. And then I found blues dancing, which was something that I could do that was exciting and very low risk and that added a lot of really meaningful relationships into my life. I've been doing it ever since; it's been a massive component in my reintegrating into society after the military.

"Prior to dancing, I was mostly just a newly returned soldier who didn't have anything to do but try to recover. Dancing was a safe space, which is something I didn't have much of prior to dance. I was looking for some sort of solace, and I found that with the dance scene. Memories from the military are more or less ever present; it's not like you can just put all that stuff in the trash. It's more a question of 'What can I do in my daily life to suspend the magical moments where those memories aren't there?' And 'How can I connect with other humans amid those memories?'"

Dancing served as the mechanism that allowed Ryan to connect with other people. On the dance floor, he didn't have to relive emotions but, rather, got a break from them. "Being able to connect with people physically, and being able to understand where they are at without talking, is really healing. That connection to other humans, that safe touch and safe space, is something that's otherwise hard to create."

Ryan gained so much through his own experience dancing that he became deeply inspired to share this outlet with others. Five years ago, he stepped into a position of leadership, as the vice president of the board for the nonprofit organization Portland Blues and Jazz Dance Society, which operates Portland's longest running weekly blues dance.

Serving on the board is not a paid position, but it's a labor of love, and work that Ryan considers very fulfilling. He invests eight hundred hours per year toward the success of the local blues dance scene. "I've taken a break from it before, but the people keep me coming back. I'd have a hard time *not* doing this work, as it gives me access to really amazing people who are very forward thinking. Being around their company helps me be more human, more grounded. The dance community is basically arms full of giant hugs, people who are radically accepting and who don't care who you are as long as you aren't disrespectful to others. Everyone is just there to dance; that is the common ground."

Ryan not only serves on the board—he further works to expand the community by occasionally teaching dance lessons before the events. "As a teacher, I want to encourage people to express themselves openly and freely without being fearful. Every time I teach a beginner lesson, I always ask, 'How many of you are afraid to be here?' and more than half of them raise their hands. I'm like, 'Well done—good for you.' It's scary, to go from never having danced, to having your friend drag you there. I think most humans have that fear, whether it be dance or public speaking or having eyes upon them."

I can attest that Ryan's presence is a calming one, however. I have seen students fall into relative ease shortly after he begins a class. Besides overcoming fear of self-expression, it's important to Ryan that he helps educate the public on what proper blues dancing is. "There's a whole misconception that it's just about 'dancing silly,' but there's actually skill to it. There's a history and tradition behind it."

When he's not running the dance, Ryan still takes time to get out on the dance floor himself. After all these years, he's still able to experience the dance high. "My favorite dance experiences are when dancing with someone to a song that neither of us has heard before, yet we have the feeling of knowing where *everything* is in the song, every hit. We are so connected, we could read each other's thoughts. After the dance, we just look at each other like 'What happened?!'"

Ten years after getting out of the military, Ryan still needs those moments to deal with the repercussions of war. "I don't feel safe talking about my military stuff often—even with people I really cherish. It feels like I'm just throwing data at you, and you're trying to understand, but you can't, and throwing data at you will not change that.

"Dancing has helped me learn so much about my place in the world. Without dance, I would not have discovered the healing power of touch or learned about different ways of living and working in the world."

Ryan's involvement with the blues scene is what led him to attend and graduate from massage therapy school. He is currently building his own massage therapy practice. "Being able to connect physically with people is really amazing. One of my biggest love languages is touch, so being a massage therapist is perfect for me. I can heal people through touch, which at the same time heals me."

Ryan doesn't want to think about what his life would be like had he not listened to his friend and attended that first night of blues dancing. Now, if Ryan were to be met with resistance from people he invites to the dance, he would give the following advice: "Check out the beginner lesson—even if it's not to attend but just to watch it—and see how many other beginners are there." And if they're still hesitant to do that? "I would do what my friend did, and put my finger on their lips and say, 'Shhh.'" Ryan laughed before adding, "If I knew them well, of course."

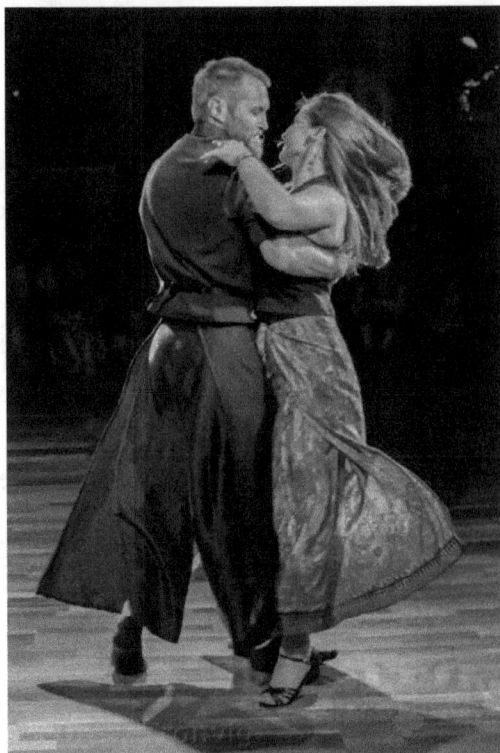

Photo by Drew Tronvig

Dancing out the Devil

Robert Grandison, London, England

"Have you met Robert yet?" Vicci, a local dance teacher and scene leader in London, asked me when I was visiting the city. "You need to meet Robert. Hold on." She glided across the room and leaned over Robert, who was seated on the patio, and wrapped her arms around his neck.

"Hey, pretty lady." He welcomed her display of affection with a pat on the hand. Robert was a strongly built, middle-aged man who spoke with a Jamaican British accent.

"Robert?" The two of them clearly had an established rapport, and Vicci knew how to use her charms. She smiled at him, doe-eyed, and spoke sweetly.

"Yes, dear?"

"Rebecca here is writing a book about the healing power of blues dancing. She's looking for people to interview who have stories of transformation. I think you should tell her your story."

Robert's casual and comfortable demeanor tightened slightly as he released a shy laugh. He appeared equal parts flattered and scared.

"You have a beautiful story. I think you should share it."

"My story, eh? Oh, I don't know."

"Here, talk to Rebecca. You two can work out the details." Vicci's smile left no room for negotiation, and she slipped away as gracefully as she had arrived.

It was my turn to put on the charm. "Well, what do you say?" I offered a sincere and, I hoped, radiant smile.

"Can we have an interview before the interview?" Robert asked.

"Sure, let's meet over tea and just get to know each other." The idea seemed to put Robert at ease. I had been met with similar reactions before—not everyone is at first comfortable with the idea of personal details being published in a book. We made plans to meet at a tube stop the following week; from there he would walk us to a place he had in mind.

The ease with which we joyfully navigated the busy streets hand-in-hand made us appear as though we were unlikely lovers. Where else, outside of the context of the dance community, could such a natural physical exchange occur across generational, racial, and gender boundaries? I wondered. We had danced together a few nights before, after Vicci had introduced us. The initial social hesitancy to engage in touch had already been broken.

Together we sat on the back patio of Wallace Collection, one of London's well-known establishments, an open roof offering a rare glimpse of sun. I'd left my notebook and recording equipment behind, since this was supposed to be just a starter conversation. I'd have to rely on memory to capture the essence of this man;

unbeknownst to him, I'd already begun taking complimentary mental notes. Though he at first appeared shy, he quickly warmed up, sharing humorous anecdotes about the city. He also already demonstrated a wealth of knowledge about British history—he'd been to the neighboring museum many times before and had several favorite pieces he was looking forward to showing me. But first, he wanted to know more about me.

"So, tell me about yourself." The interview began, but it was not me who asked the first questions. "What's your story?"

I knew that, to put him at ease, I'd be required to share some of my own journey that led me to want to write this book. I told him about how I'd been able to get over fear of touch and fear of expressing myself sensually while on the dance floor. Robert listened with interest and attentiveness. Clearly, he was a man who enjoyed connecting on a soulful level. Though he may have projected insecurity at the idea of being interviewed, he would prove to be a gifted storyteller, with a keen sense of awareness, humor, and wonder of the world.

It was well after our first cup of tea when he paused reflectively and then said, "So, my story, eh? It's probably not as dramatic as the other stories you've been hearing," he began, as nearly everyone I'd interviewed had.

"It's not drama I'm looking for," I assured him. "I'm just looking for authenticity." I knew he'd provide me with that.

"Well, about a year and half ago, my life fell apart," Robert took a moment to pause, looking down at his tea, before falling into a conversational flow. "My wife left me and walked away with most of what I'd had. I'd had huge everything—huge house, huge car, huge life. I lost it all, and just when I thought I'd hit rock bottom, she threatened that I wouldn't be able to see our two kids anymore.

"One night, it was a Friday, I was at my wit's end. I walked down the street to the Ritzy—that was my place; I intended to get drunk. I didn't know what else to do. I walked in the door and was on my way to the bar when I saw a sign that said, 'Blues,' and pointed upstairs. I didn't even see the 'dancing' part. I went up there, expecting to see a bunch of old black guys arguing about who was better, John Lee Hooker or Buddy Guy—that's what I thought I'd see. I must not have even noticed the door staff, because I didn't pay, I just walked right in, and I was shocked, I mean shocked, to see people—and *white* people at that—dancing their *hearts* out. I mean, I didn't even know what they were dancing. I couldn't tell if it was waltz or ballroom or what it was, they were dancing so wild. So I'm standing there, and this beautiful young woman comes up to me and says all sweet, 'Do you want to dance?'"

Robert paused, his eyes widening and his mouth gaping to convey the look he'd given her. The girl took that answer as a no and moved on to the next man.

"At that point, the dance organizer must have picked up on this strange new man that was throwing off the vibe of the place, and he came over and introduced himself. He invited me to join the dance, and I said, 'No, I can't dance!' But the man wouldn't take no for an answer and called over another woman to dance with me. Something in me allowed it to happen. It only took that one dance, and I already knew I wanted more.

"From then on, I started going to all the weekly classes and socials. I looked forward to the last week of the month because that meant, with the monthly dances, I could go dancing Tuesday, Thursday, Friday, and Sunday. But I didn't tell anyone what I was doing. My friends, my family, they all thought I had a woman or that I'd joined a cult or something, but then they started noticing a pattern. They'd invite me to do things on a Tuesday or Thursday, and I was always busy those nights.

"Then I started leaving the country, when I never had before. I'd go to Madrid and Berlin to dance events, but when my family asked why I was suddenly traveling so much, I'd just say, 'You wouldn't understand.' They were worried about me—I was too. I finally went to one of my teachers and said, in a whisper so no one could hear, 'All I want to do is dance. All the time. I don't understand it. Is that normal?' She laughed and called over another dancer who shared, 'All I spend my money on is dancing. Once my bills and groceries are paid, everything else goes to dance. All of it.'"

"Did you eventually tell your family what you were doing?" I asked.

"Yes, I did. I told them I was dancing to the blues, and they said, 'What?! You can't dance to blues music!' My friends, my family they still don't get it. They all think I'm crazy. You see, I never danced before. I never thought I could. But blues dancing is all about creativity and the freedom to improvise. When I discovered that—that it was improvisation that I loved—it was a big aha moment for me. I realized that was my learning style.

"I was never a good student. The academic director at the college I'd applied at pulled me aside and said, 'Before I give you your score, I have a question for you. How did you make it through year after year, for four years, when these scores reveal how stupid you are?' I answered him, 'Honestly, I don't know. But if you let me stay, I'll prove to you that I can learn.' I saw the risk. I had to learn math, or I'd get kicked out. I learned math. Now, I realize I thrive when there's a risk. I don't do well with structure, with rules. But if there's an opportunity for risk, I shine. I learned that I could apply that strength in other areas of my life. I use it now in my professional life, and I use it when I dance.

"I often ask myself: What am I doing here? Do I belong here? I mean, look at me, I'm the only black man. Why is that? I don't know what that's about. Part of me wonders if that's why I keep coming back, if I seek out opportunities where I don't belong—because there's risk in that." Robert's observation was true. Despite the inclusivity of the blues dance community, the modern scene is significantly white. I am not in a position to explain why that is, although I have observed that black culture doesn't seem to need a specified "blues dance" venue in order to dance—nor is the style of dance given that label. It's simply "dancing"—in the bar, at the backyard barbecue, or wherever the music plays and the moment is inspired.

"I'm always challenging my comfort zone now. The best dance I had last weekend was with another man. *Man,* could he follow. I mean, picture me, a heterosexual black man, dancing close embrace with another man. What is that about? I can't understand it. And yet it's completely normal. Blues dancing has stretched the boundaries in my mind of what is normal or not."

By now, we were on our third cup of tea, and the remaining water in the pot had gone cold. The chocolate croissant I'd ordered had long been picked apart, by both of us, and we were hungry. But before we gathered our belongings to move on with the day, Robert paused thoughtfully and concluded, "My ex-wife, she said the devil resided in me. Well, I don't know if that was true—to me, 'the devil' is just metaphor for the saddest time in my life. But I'm a completely different person now. I danced the devil right out of me."

Robert smiled at me, and I agreed. It might have been crooked, but there was nothing devilish about that grin.

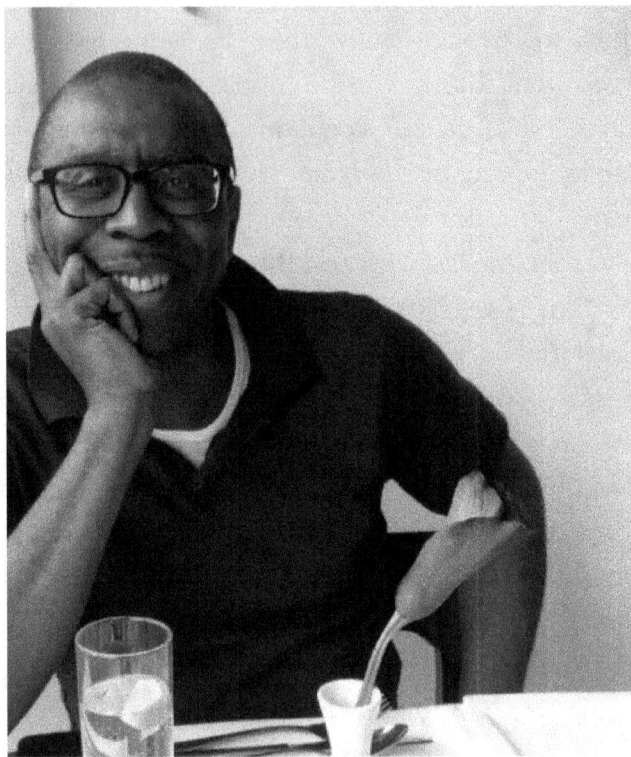

Photo by Kate Voronova

Developing My Dancer Identity

Kai Stiller, Munich, Germany

Throughout the development of this book, many moments stand out as heartwarming. One of those moments was when I received a message from Kai, a dancer I had never met before, sharing interest in contributing to this project. He began: "Right now I can give you only a glimpse of my story. It´s really hard to describe personal matters in a foreign language. Oh...and it´s really frightening too." The glimpse he gave me, however, revealed the courage that it took for him to reach out to me and made me want to know more. He shared that he was in therapy for social anxiety disorder, and that amid the near constant world of fear that he lived in, blues dancing was the anchor in his daily life.

"Sometimes, the tiny Post-it notes with dates of the next dance events are the only things that keep me going." Kai recognized the gloom that hung over such a statement and sought to reconcile the matter: "Let's try it this way: I love dancing. I do it all the time—in the kitchen, on the subway platform, in the train, on the streets. Moving to music makes me very happy. I'm excited to meet old friends again—and new people." The follow-up statement exposed a man very different from the one who began the message. As I'd come to find out, Kai considers the latter his "dancer identity." I would have the great fortune of meeting with Kai in person to hear the rest of his story when he came to Portland to attend the Waterfront Blues Festival a few months after I received his message.

We met for an informal interview at Portland's Rose Garden on a sweltering day in July; he was seated in a shady corner when I arrived. His demeanor was shy at first; I imagined he was taking in my own presence and that of the wandering tourists around us, as well as trying to find confidence speaking a foreign language. We started with the basics.

I asked Kai how he first entered the world of dance and discovered that his introduction was by no means recent. "I started ballroom dancing twenty years ago. I've always loved music—anything I can relate to that generates feelings and emotions and makes me start to move. It can be blues music, but also jazz, swing, Latin, classical." Kai found that moving to music was the easiest way for him to express himself—and also to meet other people. "All of my friends I meet through dancing. If you're shy—or anxious, in my case—then it's really hard to find a way to connect with people. Dancing is a way to say, 'This is who I am,' with just a plain question: 'Do you want to dance?'"

Kai took a break from ballroom dancing due to a jealous girlfriend, but at some point after the relationship ended, he sensed an emptiness in his personal life. He remembered that dancing had been his favorite form of therapy in the past. This time, he tried Lindy Hop, which led to an introductory class in blues. Blues moved him in a powerful way. "The complete freedom in the dance and the relationship I felt to the music blew me away. I continued with Lindy Hop for a time, but after you fall in love, you have power for only one love." Kai's eyes lit up: he had met the love of his life, in blues dance.

He began traveling overseas to satisfy his thirst to dance—preferably to live music, which was what brought him to the Portland festival. "My family knows I'm dancing and traveling a lot, and they are always telling me, 'Think about your future and save your money,' and I say no. The best way to spend my money at this moment is to spend it on dance, on meeting people. It is not something I'm throwing away. Every dollar you spend on dancing, you can remember it, because you can feel it in yourself."

Kai knows that dance is required for his well-being. "I became much more adventurous when I started dancing, and much more relaxed. To let someone come really close to you, you have to be relaxed and open." He's also become inspired by the lifestyles of the people he meets. "I've never met a blues dancer who wasn't really interesting in some way. They all do crazy stuff, like traveling all over the world just living out of their backpack, for example."

I suspect that Kai's life of dance and travel will be of great interest to many, but he doesn't see his life that way. "I have an ordinary office job. I have to push myself to travel around. I'm more of a quiet, shy person who just looks instead of talks. So when you're shy, you have to overcome some things to make dance work."

Kai started falling into a comfortable flow as he opened up to me. "My condition is called social anxiety disorder. I'm really afraid of situations with other people—even asking a clerk in a store something."

But, working with his therapist, Kai now has a tool to combat that fear. "We developed something we call 'dancer identity.' She noticed that when I talk about dancing, I'm much more confident in what I'm doing and what I'm saying. I know as well, from my experience, that I'm more confident on the dance floor, so we tried to find a way to transfer this kind of confidence into real-life situations. If there's something I think I'm not capable of doing, I imagine I'm standing on the dance floor. I think, 'Okay, I'm dancing to this song.' I have one or two specific songs to find this version of me on the dance floor: 'I'm a Man,' by Bo Diddley, and 'I'm a King Bee,' by Slim Harpo, so, really confident male songs." Kai grinned as I considered using this strategy myself, though with some strong feminine voices. "I try to transfer the confidence in the song to myself. It works sometimes—not every time, but mostly that's because I forget to think about it."

Kai has discovered other tools to help him connect with his dance partner in a way that requires confidence. "As a blues dancer in close embrace, you tend to close your eyes and feel the body connection. But what I've found makes a dance really intense is eye contact. Blues dancing with eye contact is something incredible. It completely changes the way you move.

Eyes are windows to the soul, so you give a lot away with eye contact, but you get so much back."

He considers such an experience the starting point for developing the courage to open up further. "I strongly believe you can feel the personality of someone else through dancing. If I like dancing with someone, I want to know that person better. For me, that's when I start to talk. But I can dance with people who have completely different opinions from mine, and still relate to them. There are fundamental differences between us, but dance is a way to still connect."

He has found dancing to be a way to connect with people not only of various personalities but of different ages. "I can dance with a sixty-year-old woman and have fun. Dancing is a way to communicate across generations. A grandpa can dance with his granddaughter, for example. That is a great way to connect within the family."

Kai doesn't just use dance to gain confidence in connecting with others—he uses it to access emotions and sensations within himself. After I asked what he feels when he dances, he didn't hesitate a moment before replying with conviction: "Joy. Happiness. Relaxation. After a stressful day at the office, I can go to a dance lesson after work and in just fifteen minutes forget everything that made me upset. It changes my mood really quickly. All of the positive emotions you can imagine have been generated in me through dancing."

Kai may have given up dancing for a girlfriend in the past, but he has no intention of allowing that to happen in the future. "I can't imagine a life without dancing. I don't think that's possible. I don't just dance at events with other people—I dance with myself. When I'm in the kitchen, I have music on when I'm preparing my meal. I will start wiggling my butt and shaking my hips, doing shimmies." Kai and I laughed together at the image, and I shared that I often do the same. "I can't do anything without music!"

They say, "Dance like no one's watching," but in Kai's case, he's perfected the art of dancing so that no one watching would even know that he is dancing. "There can be one hundred people around me, and they don't know it but I'm dancing. For me, it's fun to dance so no one sees it. It's kind of training for me to do these minor movements on the social dance floor. I had a friend who started to laugh when she noticed me doing tiny little shimmies in the shoulders and such. It gives you way more possibilities to express yourself—you're not just doing steps. I can stand straight in the same spot and dance with my whole body, from head to toe."

This version of Kai seems to overflow with confidence, and he's caught visual representations of his alternate personality on the dance floor as well. As Kai shared, you have to really want to change or no amount of therapy is going to work. He wants change—and, gratefully, he has found the right tool for him.

"I had a session with my therapist when I showed her four photos of me. There were two photos

158

where someone else was the focal point, but I could be seen in the background. In one of these two photos, my eyes were on something else in the room, not on the person who was talking. In the other photo, there are things happening around me, but I'm sitting by a window and looking outside. These two photos revealed what part of my problem is—I'm sometimes not very present in the room. But you have to be present to smile at other people or look friendly so that someone wants to talk to you.

"In the other two photos, I had my dancing face on, and I was so much happier. I have an expression on my face that is so relaxed, and I have this tiny little smile. It was these photos that led my therapist to change her approach with me—to develop the idea of my dancer identity."

His therapist has remarked on the progress Kai has made in overcoming his fear through the use of this tool. "She said she's really proud of me. I'm afraid of social contact, yet I do social dancing and travel to social dances. Those are things you wouldn't expect from someone who's afraid of people. But I do it, and she said that's incredible. Dancing gives me the strength and the courage to do it. If you're doing social dance, you have to socialize with other people—there's just no way around it."

It's a predicament he has chosen to accept, over and over again—and one that he encourages others who struggle with the same fears he does to pursue themselves. "To someone else who has social anxiety, I would give the advice to go to a class with someone you know and trust. And I would say listen to music at home and dance to it. There's a documentary about treating Alzheimer's patients with music called *Alive Inside*. They play music from their youth, and suddenly they start to open their eyes—you can reach them through music. Music and dance can change your life…and *keep* you alive. If life gets you down, if you're angry or something, just remember you can turn on some tunes and start to move. It's a way to forget everything and find another mood." Or even find a whole new identity.

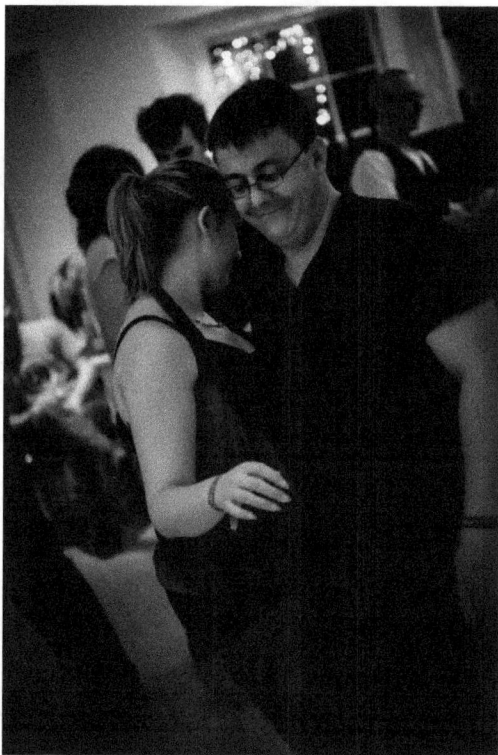

Photo by Jelena Lihhatsova (Fair City Blues)

The Making of Me

Lorna, Hertfordshire, England

Lorna came across this book project shortly after she'd made a declaration of her own transformation through blues dancing on her local dance scene's online social forum. She wondered if it was serendipity; she contacted me, directing me to her recent post, and I followed up for more of her story.

One of the neatest parts about this project for me is all of the lovely people I've gotten to meet—even if not yet in person. My list keeps growing of thoughtful, open-hearted people to follow up with when I'm in this country or that. I feel honored to be trusted with such personal insight into the worlds of people like Lorna.

Lorna doesn't usually share the intimate parts of her life with friends—let alone strangers—unless they are a part of the blues dance community. As has already been shared by other contributors to this book, blues dancers just seem more willing to go "there." And "there" is a place Lorna increasingly feels called to go.

Her story began after her twenty-year marriage ended. A friend saw how consumed Lorna had become with work and raising her two children and felt she needed to do "something for herself for once."

The first dance she went to was a rock/modern jive dance. It clicked instantly for Lorna. "I danced all evening, I couldn't sleep that night. I thought, 'Oh my goodness! Men can dance!' It felt so amazing; I can't explain it. I actually had to travel four hours the next day at six in the morning, and I can remember having not slept."

What most intrigued Lorna was that social dancing was a safe place to socialize. She wasn't looking for love, but she did want to meet new people.

Lorna attended numerous classes—one of which ended up being a blues taster. She instantly connected with the freedom to express herself in a nonprescripted way.

"My whole life is about control—no one can organize like I can. But I started to really love dancing, because I didn't have to do that. I wasn't Ms. Organize anymore. I just did what someone else told me to do, for the first time in my life!" Lorna laughed "I quite liked it. I had no responsibility, and I got all the enjoyment."

About a year after the taster class, Lorna booked a boot camp blues workshop for two days. Lorna's first impression at the camp was that everyone was really friendly. However, at lunchtime on the first day, she nearly went back home. "I was in tears. I was overcome with the thought, 'This is too hard. I can't do it.' I thought I had made a huge mistake. I'm a perfectionist, and I felt I wasn't able to do things right."

Lorna stuck with it, though, and it only got better. "By the end of the day, I was on cloud nine. It started to come together when we danced freestyle. I thought, 'Maybe I can do this!' I intended to leave after the workshop on Sunday, but I ended up staying until 11:00 p.m.!'"

When she got home, she reflected on what she'd just done. "I was like, 'Oh my goodness, I've just been wiggling my hips in front of people!'" Lorna and I laughed together, but the significance of that experience held great depth. "For the first time ever, I let my inhibitions go. I'd done something for me, not for anyone else, and didn't feel guilty."

Lorna continued her exploration of blues dancing. She attended another blues boot camp later that year. The same insecurities arose at first: "There was that learning curve again, where I felt like I couldn't do it. But then on the second day, the teacher did something really amazing. She split the group into men and women, and with the women she had us focus on the idea of letting go—being led, going with the flow, and listening closely to the music. When we got back together with the men to practice together, the song 'Let Her Go,' by Passenger, was played. I danced with this guy I'd never danced with before, and I just let him lead the dance. When the song ended, we grouped together again for the teacher to talk to us, and I thought, 'I'm going to cry.' I couldn't hold the emotion in, and I looked over at my dance partner, and *he* was crying! He later commented that the dance we had was one of the best he'd ever had and one that he'd never forget." Clearly, it was one she would never forget, either.

Lorna has since gotten more and more comfortable accessing her emotions. For most of her life, she was deeply concerned with what she looked like and what others thought of her. But dancing has allowed her opportunities to set those concerns behind.

"I actually get therapy out of dancing. In the UK, we don't do 'real' therapy—there's this mindset that seeing a therapist is something you do when you've failed. But all I need is dancing to put me in a good place.

"It's something I do for me. I think there are people who don't need 'me' time, but I need to keep my identity. Having been in a marriage for twenty years where I lost my identity, I don't want to go back to that. I am still a mum, partner, and work colleague, but dancing has given me my own identity as well, which has greatly enriched my life."

Lorna is in a new relationship now, with a partner who doesn't dance, but he understands and supports her love for it.

"He came to watch me for the first time last October, and he didn't have a problem, but I did." Lorna offered a shy, guilty smile. "I couldn't dance! We were staying in a hotel overnight, and he said, 'I'm going to go back to the hotel, but I want you to stay and enjoy yourself.' He doesn't have any qualms about me dancing, because he understands that it's my passion, and that I come home to him. I'm very lucky in that respect. But to me, it's not about sexuality and fear that someone is going to find me attractive—it's that finally I feel attractive to myself.

"Before, if someone told me I look really nice, I would have said, 'Yeah, but my hair is not right'—that's how I always used to answer a compliment. I remember a friend of mine saying to me, 'All you have to do is say thank you.' So I practice that now. I give compliments out more now too.

"I had no self-esteem, and I have this little ego thing that tells me that everything I do is wrong. Helping me break out of that pattern is what dancing has been able to do for me. I never used to wear dresses or sleeveless tops, and now I've got so many dress shoes it's unbelievable," Lorna giggled like a teenage girl. "But I don't do it for anyone else but me."

Dancing has entered her role as a mother, as well. "I listen to a lot more music now, and my little boy loves it. I'll put some music on, and we'll just be dancing around. For him, my dancing actually makes him more open-minded and not embarrassed to be silly. If we're walking down the street, I'll do a twirl with him, and he just loves it.

"I'm much more confident overall. I worry less about things, and I worry less about what people think of me. I still am a perfectionist, but now I think it's great when I don't finish something, or when I decide that if something isn't for me then I won't pursue it to the end because that's what you should do."

She's also more likely to stand up for herself at work. "I'm a more confident person overall because of dancing. Before, I would think that my input wasn't very relevant, or no one's going to listen to it. But now I feel more assured that my views are just as valid as anybody else's. I can even walk into a room full of people at a social venue by myself now—that's a major step for me."

Lorna goes out dancing as much as she can—but she recognizes it's not what has to come first in her life. "Dancing has to fit in around everything else. It has to play a part, but it can't come before anything else. But I think that keeps everything in context for me, and it probably means that I enjoy it more because I don't get as much of it, so I savor what I get.

"Had I not found it at all, however, my life would have been very different. I feel that dancing was the missing piece in my journey, and now that I have it, I feel the best I ever have about myself."

Our interview was kept to a defined duration—mom duties called. But as Lorna said good-bye, the energy with which she moved carried a proper sense of purpose. She emitted the essence that she was not just a mom but a woman unto herself.

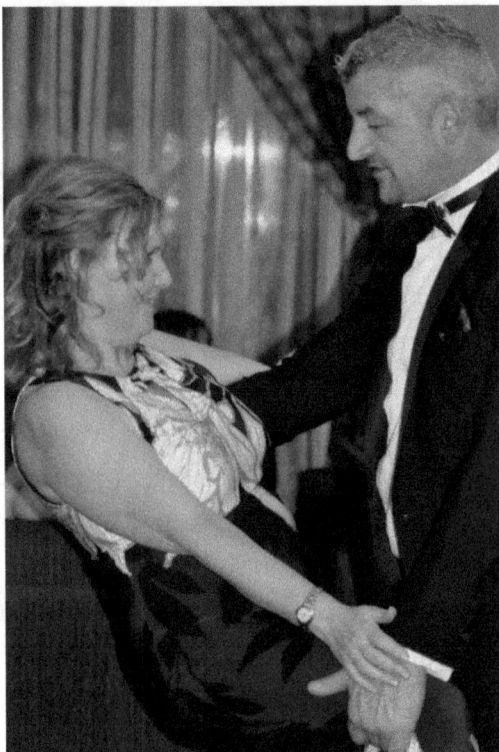

Photo by Sara White

IV
SOUL

Several of the people interviewed in this book spoke of how modern culture has become almost entirely cerebral. The arts—and physical education, for that matter—have been entirely eliminated from many schools, considered secondary to math and sciences and SAT scores. As a result, we have become more and more removed from the soul—from forces within us and in the universe that can't be seen or scientifically explained.

Various tools or creative outlets can remind us, however. For the people in this section, dance has been the instrument of choice to bring them into contact with their inner worlds, or with a spirit world. A particular religion or faith does not have to be practiced in order for one to be able to access the soul. The dancers in this section come from highly varied spiritual backgrounds: Christianity, Buddhism, Hinduism, Taoism, and even atheism. Yet all of them can attest to being able to access a sensation much bigger than themselves…while dancing the blues.

Some of these individuals had to work through conflict between faith and the dance floor. They may have needed to question or alter their perception of what it meant to practice their particular religion in order to fully express themselves. But in the end, it was blues dancing that brought them out of their minds, even out of their bodies—and into their souls.

If Jesus Were Here, He'd Be Dancing at a Blues Bar

Jana Jade, Nashville, Tennessee, USA

Women don't typically meet other women in the partner dance world. At least, that has been my experience. There's a risk to extending a greeting to another woman waiting to be asked to dance. I don't often do this because it means I'll be in conversation and therefore unavailable to dance. I'd rather dance.

But sometimes situations call for taking that risk. I spent a few months last spring in Nashville, Tennessee, a city I once lived in. I arrived alone at the Bourbon Street Blues and Boogie Bar downtown. Stepping inside what was once a second home to me, I noticed a corner table that seemed to be where the local blues dancers congregated—dancers can be easily spotted by their dance shoe bags, their mounds of belongings, and their chairs pushed aside to maximize dance floor space.

Eight years after I'd lived there, I no longer knew anyone there. But out of the group, one particular woman caught my eye. Her essence was that of a modern Southern belle; she was beautiful in multiple senses of the word. She carried herself with poise, and there was a charming, sweet nature about her—oh, and that Southern drawl.

I was instantly intimidated. I didn't grow up in the South; I'd lived there for a few years, but I grew up in Wisconsin, and I still felt my tom-girl roots radiating in stark contrast to the woman that stood before me. I have learned, however, that the best way to dispel intimidation is to face it head on. "Hi, I'm Rebecca." I smiled and introduced myself. "Hi! I'm Jana. And this is my mom." Jana turned to the woman seated behind her, who extended a warm hello. Not many people bring their moms to a blues dance. I started to feel less intimidated and a bit more intrigued.

That one greeting led to a lengthy conversation that evolved from the standard "Where are you from?" and "How long have you been blues dancing?" to the mutual realization that we were both women in our early thirties, raised conservative Christian, who had found healing from sexual repression and shame through blues dancing. I did not see *that* conversation coming within the first few minutes of meeting someone—especially just after I'd been introduced to her mom. We felt a mutual desire to continue talking, off the dance floor. We agreed to meet for coffee the following week, and I was delighted to find that she was enthusiastic about sharing her story for this book.

Jana was a recent Nashville transplant. She had grown up in the tiny community of Warthen, Georgia. Even though she left at the age of eighteen to attend college in Atlanta, she said she never really left Warthen in her heart—and she never had to "grow up," until she moved to Nashville, which wouldn't happen for another decade. While in Atlanta, she married her college sweetheart—a man she'd known since high school. Her life plans seemed to be falling into place; she pictured herself having kids before long and had already established a savings account to prepare for the day her parents needed support. She was proud of her accomplishments. But there was one missing detail—her marriage was falling apart. Divorce had not been part of her plan—nor was it in agreement with her faith.

"I grew up very conservative Christian. I checked all the boxes, did everything by the book, so to speak. Having premarital sex was very taboo, so I tried to avoid that, which is probably why I got married so young." Jana was married for nine years before divorce became imminent.

Upon hearing the official news, her brother came and got her and encouraged her to join him on a cross-country road trip. What she never would have agreed to in the past, Jana said yes to without hesitation. She knew she needed a fresh start. Jana headed West—with plans to settle in Nashville at the end of her return journey.

When we met, she'd been in Nashville for only a few months, but she was glowing with happiness. She hadn't yet started working, and the luxury of time allowed her to process the turn her life had taken. "This is the longest I've ever gone without a job. Thankfully, I had a good amount of savings due to my lifestyle before—I had put off everything for this future, this plan of a house on the hill, a family, moving back home next to my parents, taking care of them. I realized that I'd put off a lot of current happiness for the future— which was good in a way, because I did have this cushion for when my marriage ended, but at the same time, it made me realize how those behaviors were probably affecting my marriage."

When Jana returned to Nashville, she knew she would need the help of a professional to access those patterns she'd overlooked before. She started seeing a therapist who told her, "Jana I think the best thing that ever happened to you is your life falling apart." Jana admitted, "That was hard to hear at the time, but I've started to learn to accept that and realize she's right. I'd stopped growing. I'd completely stopped bringing other people into my life because I had this thought that if it's temporary, if it's impermanent, why even make the effort?" If a relationship wasn't contributing to her ultimate goal of moving back to Warthen near her family, Jana wanted no part of it.

By the time we spoke, she had realized that that way of thinking actually went against the religion she was so desperately trying to follow. "There's scripture about not hiding your light—not putting your light under a bushel—and there I was, isolating myself from other human beings. Yes, I had my acquaintances at work, but other than my family, that was it." Jana looked across the table at me and realized even this moment would never have happened had she kept those beliefs.

"I wouldn't have gone to coffee with you during those years. I would have thought, 'What's the point? She doesn't live here, so why get attached to her?' That's the wrong attitude to have in life, because it doesn't matter how long someone's in your life—if it's for a few seconds, a few weeks, or a few years, they bring something to your life."

The passion behind Jana's newfound conviction was evident in the speed at which her thoughts began to roll into spoken words, and in the eye contact she maintained to display just how present she was with me.

"Now I see the beauty in the moment and in impermanence. And I realize that I'm never alone. Even though we feel alone sometimes, a lot of people feel the same way we do. We are connected. That's the one thing that keeps coming back to me all the time—this understanding of our connection to the light of God and the light in other people that we come across."

Her words harkened back to what I'd heard others describe in earlier interviews, so I was not surprised when Jana began to share that it was dancing that helped lead her to that appreciation of the present moment. "I can remember the date—it's almost like someone remembering the date of her baptism." Jana laughed. "My friend Lauren from church mentioned that she did swing dancing on Friday nights. I thought that sounded like fun, and since I wasn't really doing anything Friday or Saturday nights—I just kind of sat at home—I figured, why not try it? I'd always enjoyed dancing growing up, but I'd never really found my niche in it.

"So I went with her, and there was a lesson where they taught us East Coast Swing, but then when they turned down the lights, a guy came over to ask me to dance. I was really nervous, but I just looked into his eyes and smiled. We started dancing, and I didn't know what he was doing, but I knew I liked it, and then finally I realized that his type of dancing was really different from the type of dancing that everyone else was doing. I liked his better."

What he was dancing was blues. And it brought her to another world.

"Dancing was almost like heaven for me in my imagination, in that you never turned anybody down. You would dance with every person and learn something from each one of them. It felt like falling in love over and over again."

Jana was invited to go dancing the following night at Whiskey Bent Saloon, a honky-tonk bar on lower Broadway. She went, and got invited to go dancing the night after that at another venue. Suddenly her social calendar was packed. And she attended blues workshops, blues house parties, and blues lessons before the monthly dances.

"I made some good friends really quickly just being in the blues classroom. I thought, 'Okay, all of the people I've met through dance have been really nice, but there's something really special about the blues group. And there's something special about the style. There's this freedom in blues to do whatever you want, move however you feel, and yes, it works best when you're in connection with your partner, but there's also a freedom to do your own thing as well."

Even a year ago, blues dancing would not have been okay in Jana's book. "Even when a mushy scene would be on the TV, I would look away. I never showed a lot of public affection even with my husband, and I would judge other people if they showed affection with theirs. I didn't start dating until I was out of high school. I remember my dad asking my mom, 'Are our daughters "all right"? Because they're not dating at all.'"

When Jana was ready to start dating, she told herself she didn't even want to kiss anyone unless she was going to marry him. The first person that she ever kissed was, in fact, her husband. "I thought that because we did everything 'right,' we were going to be together till the end."

At the time of our interview, the end of her marriage was recent enough for her emotions around the situation to still be raw. "Part of me still struggles with it. I never thought I'd be in this position. Basically, this is my worst nightmare, but at the same time I realize that the way I was living my life wasn't healthy. I had to lose him to learn that. And it was all worth it, because at least as I move forward in my life, I will live truly and genuinely. I won't be hiding and not connecting with other people."

Jana is grateful to have found an outlet for connecting with others through dancing—and also an outlet to explore her femininity and sexuality in a way she'd never allowed herself to do before. "I always had issues as a female, not feeling very feminine. So after our relationship ended—and since he'd cheated on me—I didn't feel desirable or attractive. Once I got into dancing, it made me tap into that part of myself."

This led me to recall the first night I'd met Jana, when she'd introduced me to her mom. To bring her mom to a blues dance seemed to be a sign that Jana was not just tapping into her femininity but displaying it for others. I asked her what her mom's impression was of that night at the blues bar. "She was very nervous just to be there in the first place, so I ordered her a blue drink," Jana laughed. "We wore blue dresses for the blues dance and drank blue drinks, and you know, after that she just said she really enjoyed watching me. She said that I looked so happy and free out there. I'm so glad I can share that part of myself with her, because I want my family to see where I've found joy."

With Jana's exploration of herself has come an exploration of her faith. I was reminded of the Buddhist proverb, "When the student is ready, the teacher appears," as Jana spoke of an unexpected friendship she had recently developed.

"I met this seventy-one-year-old Jewish-Buddhist man while dancing at Dance World. I call him Mr. Larry, and he is a student of life. We had this long conversation after we danced, and from there we started meeting on Fridays for coffee and interfaith dialogue. I come from a very evangelistic Christian background, so I need to be really aware of myself when I have these discussions. Otherwise, I go back to that preset 'Jesus Christ is the Lord, John 14:6 ("I am the way and the truth and the life. No one comes to the Father except through me"),' and I stop fully listening."

Jana's conversations with Mr. Larry were not her first exposure to Buddhism, but she finds herself more open now to considering the application of some of its principles into her own life. "My first experience with Buddhism was in college in my Religion 101 class. I realized that even if it didn't feel like a religion for me, it was a good way to live one's life. I am still Christian, but I've taken things I like from Buddhism and brought them into my life."

When I asked her for some examples of this practice, she had several to offer.

"I love the concept in Buddhism of right mindfulness—being really present and in the moment. I have moments where I'm dancing with someone, and I realize that my mind is wandering. I try to always bring myself back to the dance, because the person I'm dancing with is important, and I need to appreciate that and be fully present with him.

"It's helped me in other avenues of life too. Even just walking past a person, just acknowledging that that's a human being and that might be the only time that I cross his or her path on this planet. But one day, in my faith, we will all be up there dancing together." Jana gestured toward the sky.

No matter one's faith, I believe that's a beautiful picture to imagine.

Jana brought the conversation back to her evangelical background. These days, she proselytizes a different sort of tenet. "I feel almost like I've become a dance evangelist because I try to invite everybody into dancing!" Jana laughed at herself. "I'm just so excited about it. I might meet somebody in line at the store— usually single women—and it will just come up in conversation. If they are not having a good day, I'll tell them, 'You should go dancing!'"

Her neck swayed, and her hand raised as she declared, "People get really judgy about blues dancing and shaking your hips, but guess what. If Jesus were here now, he'd be dancing at a blues bar."

I allowed that image to playfully reside in my mind before Jana continued, "Going out dancing at night is spiritually, emotionally, and physically just a healthier way to live. Finding dance when I did has really helped me transition from all the hurt that I've experienced. I'm still grieving, but it's given me an outlet to work with that grief and move forward. I can accept the beauty in grief now. Even in failure there's beauty, and you can go on from that. Dance teaches you that it's okay to let go of control. Things happen. You might fall down or bump into somebody, but you can just start back over on the beat."

It's true. Whether it's the beat of life or the beat of the music—if we listen for it, we can always start back over.

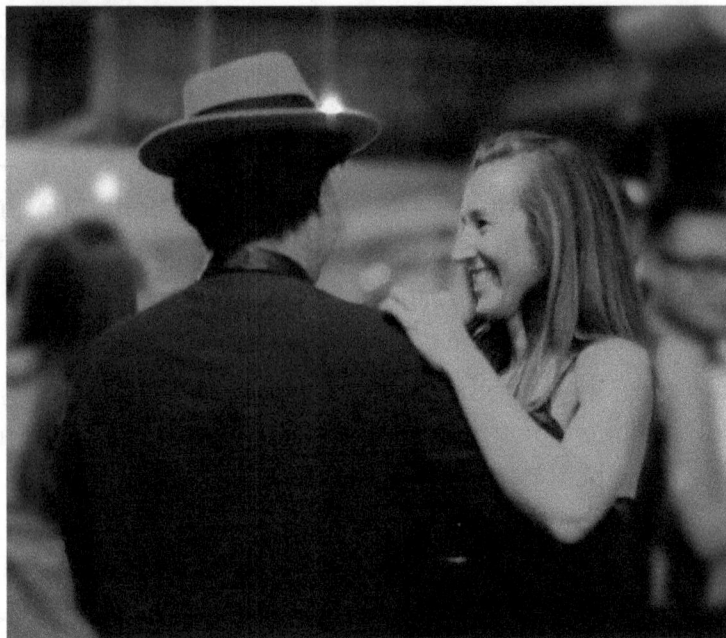
Photo by Yugandhar Beesetty

The Tantra of the Blues

Jenny Lynn, Great Dunmow, England

Jenny interviewed me before I interviewed her. Through the social media world, she found out about this book project—and, therefore, the previous book I'd written, and invited me to share my story on her therapy practice's podcast. My story of having overcome fear of sexual expression through dancing the blues was what led Jenny to call me "a woman after her own heart." Her professional work is dedicated to helping others overcome the same, and her own transformation through blues dancing has inspired her to want to share this particular tool with her clients.

Jenny operates her own business as a practitioner of transpersonal therapy, or therapy that "goes beyond the personality into the heart of the client." She also recently became a tantra practitioner, what she described as "working spiritually with the body through mindfulness and breath." Tantra is most often associated in the Western world as a sexual practice—which Jenny affirms it can be, but it doesn't have to be.

For example, she described that you could be having a tantric experience if you are drinking a glass of water and are aware of every single aspect of that experience—that you're holding a glass; that when you raise it to your lips, there is coolness in your mouth; that you can feel the sensation of the water entering your body. In dance, this means being aware of the music on a very minute level, or of your partner's breath, or of every physical point of connection between you—as well as energetic and emotional.

By paying deeper attention to all of our senses, we are paving a path for growth, Jenny believes. "Dancing is really personal development. Blues dancing is more than dancing. It's not just about the moves; it's about how it feels to move. When you move the body, how does that move the mind? How does it move your soul? If the body and the mind and the soul are one, how does that feel? Let's get into the tantra of it; let's get into how it feels right now to be at one with yourself."

It took Jenny many years before she felt not only at one with herself but in a position to share with others how she came to these understandings. Her journey is one she felt uncomfortable sharing with the larger world, deeming it inappropriate to reveal in her profession. However, in the last few years, Jenny has gone from not only owning her story among family and friends but proudly sharing it on her professional website.

I asked her to tell me more about the mental health crisis in her twenties that led her to pursue her current line of work. She began, "During a period of extreme stress, I was more or less sleepless for many months. Eventually I started to be unable to organize my thoughts." She was subsequently diagnosed with schizophrenia.

"Schizophrenia is a state of mind that I would call a parallel reality. In it, you see and perceive things in a different order of magnitude to the average person's version of reality. There is a lot of fear in schizophrenia. You are alone with your insights and thoughts."

Jenny was already on the path to a healthier self before dance entered into the picture. In the couple of tumultuous years before her schizophrenic episode, Jenny had met Buddhism. In the depths of her schizophrenia, she found herself chanting almost involuntarily, as though there were some greater but unconscious motive. It was a few years later she had an epiphany: she realized that trying to fix patterns in her life were dependent on entering into a higher level of consciousness, or awareness. Being fully present in the here and now was the only way to be "awake." Now in her fifties, she has discovered another more interactive and fun way of practicing mindfulness—through dancing the blues.

After a lifelong interest in dance, Jenny was introduced to what is known in the UK as modern jive a few years ago, which led her to blues dancing. She attended a one-day blues dance workshop, where she had a dance that rivaled the connection she has been able to experience in her tantric practice. "There was a moment of looking into my partner's eyes, and it was like I knew who he was. I could see what he's been through; I could see his suffering; I could see his dissonance, his passion for dance. It was almost like there was no screen between us, no filter. I saw him. I don't know if he saw me, but I certainly saw him. For that three or four minutes, we were part of each other. We were able to move in unison so easily, because there had been that spiritual and emotional connection. I'd never had that experience on the dance floor before. It was electrifying, that you can have that level of intensity for the three and a half minutes that it takes to have a dance."

Soon after, Jenny attended a blues event and had another epiphany. "I was watching people dance, and I saw what was possible. I saw what the potential was with blues. I was witnessing before my eyes the most exotic, inspiring dance movements, and I was transfixed. That event gave me complete permission to be myself on the dance floor—to explore the rhythms, to explore the movement, to really interpret the music in any way I wanted. It was a freedom, a casting off."

Since that night, Jenny has evolved into a woman her friends hardly recognize. "I was dancing last weekend, and several of my dance friends said, 'Jenny, look at you—you're not the same person that you were a year ago.' It's true—I've lost a lot of weight; I've vamped up my appearance; I'm really comfortable in my skin."

Now, she is on a mission to inspire others to be as comfortable in their bodies as she has become, and she's doing it by using blues dance techniques in her therapy workshops. "In addition to my private therapy sessions, I also run workshops called Clear the Fear. I was incorporating bits of movement into my workshops before, but they weren't big movements. But I recently ran an event exploring Clear the Fear of Intimacy, and I introduced a few exercises that I've learned from the blues—starting with just gaining confidence wiggling your shoulders or your hips." The strategy worked with her students, and Jenny became inspired to develop her teaching skills to implement this technique on a deeper level.

"I attended traditional blues workshops and classes and watched quite a few videos on YouTube. Then I went to Prague, and I trained to be a blues dance teacher, and now I'm voraciously gobbling up every snippet of interpretation movement lessons that I can and incorporating them into my own ideas about how to teach the blues. To be on the dance floor with someone you can connect with and express yourself with and explore a moment of oneness with is one of the most beautiful gifts you could ever offer someone as a dance teacher, as a mentor, or as a workshop leader."

Jenny is now teaching blues dancing in her local town, outside of her therapy practice. "I really want to spread the word. I would love a world where people are at one in their bodies and happy in their skin. They know how to own their feelings and their thoughts and are honest and genuine and at one with themselves. And I think the movements of the blues teach that."

Blues dancing taught her that lesson; she no longer wishes to hide any part of herself. "It's taken a while, but I've had to accept that I'm an unusual person." Jenny laughed. "I didn't want to be unusual. I wanted to be accepted in my profession, and I did everything possible to hide my unusualness, but it just seeped through. What's happened in the last few years is my schizophrenia story has seeped out of me. I had to start sharing it because it's such a unique story, to recover from something that the majority of the world says you don't recover from."

Jenny believes it was her spiritual path that led her to that realization first, but it was blues dancing that led her to embody it. "I've been on this Buddhist journey for more than thirty years but only truly moving into my body in the last few years through this whole tantric blues movement." And contrary to her initial fear, being completely authentic about her past and her practices hasn't damaged her professional credibility—but rather, in some instances, heightened it.

"A client said the other day that when she read my story on my website, she thought, 'If you can heal you, then I'm sure you can heal me.' So I've got nothing to hide, nothing to be ashamed of. I think now is the time to not hide. Now is the time to be known. The way forward in all of our lives is to share stories. We need more storytellers." Jenny paused thoughtfully before adding with a smile, "And more dancers."

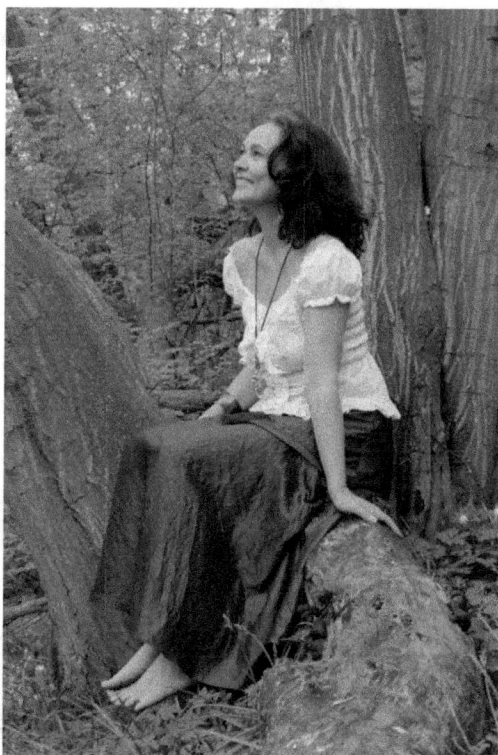

Photo by Pete Gowing

Meditating with a Partner

Krunal Waghela, Mumbai, India

Blues dancers often have a curious relationship with Lindy Hop dancing. As demonstrated throughout this book, it is typical to discover blues dancing via a circuitous route that began with Lindy Hop. For many, blues hence becomes one's preferred dance style—but especially because Lindy Hop is more mainstream than blues, even die-hard blues lovers may attend Lindy Hop events from time to time.

Such was the case for Krunal and me; we met at the 2013 London Lindy Exchange. When the band experimented with a slower blues-like number, in the midst of the more typical up-tempo jazz numbers, I saw the dancers alter their jazz steps to the new beat simply by slowing them down. I was not interested in jazz steps. I wanted to throw down proper *blues* moves. And, apparently, so did Krunal.

"Do you dance blues?"

The accent sounded perhaps Indian—I opened my eyes from my trance state to see a man looking back at me with some hesitation.

"Yes," I replied, with what must have been a look of deep hope. "Do you?"

His response was pure elation. "Yes!" In a room full of over four hundred bouncing Lindy Hop dancers, we'd found our ideal dance partners—covert blues aficionados, the both of us.

Though we have not seen each other since that event, at the time of this interview two years later, Krunal remembers that moment as clearly as I do. "It was this wonderful thing, a blues song being played when I saw you. I was like, 'This looks like a blues person.' Somehow it shows up in the personality—there's something in the face that says, 'This is a blues dancer.'"

Krunal had lived in the United States for several years—where he first learned to dance—but was traveling around the United Kingdom at the time we met. He has since moved back to his native Mumbai, India, where in addition to his career in engineering, he has taken it upon himself to spread the love of dancing through teaching blues and Lindy Hop classes. "I felt a desire to give back to the world what I had experienced in the US and UK when I went dancing. People gave me so much love, so much positivity, even though I did not know them."

That love and positivity came at a time when Krunal really needed it. Having moved to the United States for his studies in engineering, Krunal had very little time for socializing until he neared graduation in 2009. "I started looking for a full-time job in my industry at that time. However, there was a recession in the US economy, making my search difficult. I had a lot of time and didn't know what to do with it, so I decided to check out the recreation center for the first time."

Krunal's campus recreation center, in addition to martial arts, aerobics, and other sports, also offered an aerial swing dance club, which piqued his interest for a couple of reasons. "I was never into dancing. I was too intimidated. I felt it was something I couldn't do. I always like to challenge myself, so I said okay, if it doesn't work out, I won't go again."

Aside from a personal challenge, Krunal had another motive. "Girls usually like men who dance," he laughed. "I thought, someday I'm going to have my girlfriend or my wife, and she could be someone who likes to dance. I didn't want to be the guy who can't dance. I would want to be able to dance with her to bring her joy and happiness."

Krunal gave the class a try and was surprised by the result. "Before, I didn't understand why someone would dance, but it was a whole different thing when I experienced it. There is a connection and exchange of energy that happens with the other person—and not just with your partner but with other people dancing around you—that was something I'd never thought about before. I realized, dancing was a creative outlet for me."

Krunal started traveling to attend dance events, which exposed him to new people and new dance styles. While attending a swing social event at a university in Columbia, Missouri, he discovered blues music and dancing for the first time. "I couldn't figure out if it was swing music or not. It sounded different, but I didn't know why. And then I saw this couple dancing to a different footwork. It was really slow and passionate and smooth. It was not bouncy like swing; it was very nice to watch. I thought, 'This might be something I'd like to try next.'"

After moving to Washington D.C. upon acquiring an engineering role there, Krunal began attending a weekly blues dance class and found that the style fit more with his personality. "I'm very deep inside. I tend to think a lot and move slowly. I am patient; I don't make decisions in a hurry." Blues quickly became his favorite style of dance—one in which he was able to connect not only with his own personality but with the soul of another.

"Usually meditation is by yourself, but when you're dancing blues, it is like meditating with a partner. There's a connection beyond the physical. I think the souls can connect for a few minutes together. It doesn't matter who I'm dancing with—within the body there is this energy of two people blending together, trying to understand each other."

Krunal described meditation as "a very deep state of mind, body and soul where my awareness level is raised so high that nothing else matters around me. I forget who I am, what is happening in my life, I forget any worries or problems I have. This state allows one to connect with the inner self; to channel energy to our essential requirements only, of happiness, peace and bliss."

Such an experience is what has led some people to say, "Blues is my religion"—acclaimed American blues musician Sonny Rhodes even wrote a song by that title—but Krunal has another religion; he is a practicing

Hindu. Although Krunal has used blues dancing as a tool to enhance his religion's meditation practice, there are other cultural barriers he has had to overcome with his students in order to perceive the dance as respectable.

"Close embrace with strangers is not typical in Indian culture, similar to many other cultures around the world. Hence, many people who are used to social dancing are not often open to dancing blues in close embrace." Although blues doesn't have to be in close embrace, Krunal and I agreed that if it is avoided completely, the dance is significantly limited in scope.

"I'm trying to explain to people that dancing blues in close embrace doesn't necessarily mean anything wrong. I tell them it is just a dance—all you have to worry about is leading or following and enjoying the dance with that person for those three to four minutes. If you fall in love with that person, just keep it in those three to four minutes." Krunal laughed, aware that this is an experience that does sometimes occur on the dance floor. "Unless you really, *really* connect, of course. That's different."

Krunal also makes a point to teach social etiquette in his classes. "When I teach blues, I tell them there are things you can do to avoid uncomfortable situations. If something doesn't go right, there are ways you can work around it. You are not forced to be in close embrace, which is something they have to understand. When they do understand that, they are willing to give it a try."

It's a tall order Krunal is taking on, to change what has been the ingrained culture around dance, but a shift has been taking place over the past few years to help him with his mission. With globalization, people in India are being exposed to bachata, Argentine tango, and kizomba—all close-embrace dances. Krunal believes that many people who are open to these close embrace dances would also be open to exploring blues. "Usually when people start dancing, quite a few of them start with Lindy Hop and move on to blues. I am trying to create a strong Lindy scene now, and hopefully a strong blues scene in the future."

If anyone can develop a new scene, I believe Krunal can. He has already done a great job at laying a foundation for Lindy Hop in Mumbai. "There was no Lindy scene here before I started teaching. There were two traveling instructors who came to India and held a couple of workshops a few years ago, but there was no established scene or awareness of what Lindy Hop really was.

"The scene has grown quite a bit since I started about nine months ago. I felt it was a good idea to start teaching not just Lindy Hop but various partner dance forms. That way, people would come to me for waltz or salsa or another prominent style that people are really looking for in India, and from there I could invite them to Lindy and blues."

Krunal's family reacted optimistically about his involvement with dance. "I don't think anyone in my family is into dancing. When I was in the US and started dancing, they were like, 'What? *You* go dancing?!' But they think it's wonderful. They really like that I'm doing something I was not comfortable with, and now I'm teaching it, so they think that's a great thing. And they really like follows being all around me." We laughed at the reference to his parents' desire for him to marry.

Krunal will tell you that he first felt a heart-and-soul connection to blues dancing because of the dance itself, but it's no longer only the embrace or the pace or the people he meets that make Krunal love blues. It's the music. "The music is very deep. I can feel the pain in it."

At the time in his life when Krunal found blues, he could relate to that discomfort. "Me being a foreigner in the US, having been born and bred in India where the traditional culture is quite different, there was always this line I had to break to be one with people. I had to really try to understand them, embrace them, and be like them. Blues dancing was something that really changed my energy. I could forget the difficult part of my life and just be happy, just be in bliss, even though there was so much going on around me."

Krunal found that blues dancing also helped him understand the American culture better, allowing him to blend in more easily with people. "Dance was one common point I had with the other people around, so it made it easier to make friends from there."

It wasn't only an emotional or social experience that contributed to Krunal's healing through the blues— it was a principle he described as spiritual: "Any kind of sound or music has a frequency—there is a vibration in the air that comes in a sequence. When you hear these sounds in a particular rhythm or sequence, it has a particular effect on your body."

He continued, "As human beings, we each have our own vibration or frequency, so something that could influence me may not influence you the same way. However, there are certain frequencies that can influence a lot of different particles, or people, in a similar fashion. These frequencies can heal people—like the sound therapy people do these days—which is not any different from the healing that can happen through blues music."

The law of vibration, the scientific description for what Krunal first knew as spiritual principle, offers that healing can take place through sound alone. But Krunal suggested that adding physical contact with another human being takes it to another level. "Being alone with the music has a different healing effect than being with another person, because now there are three different energies interacting together. The healing effect is much stronger than without one of those elements being present. There's a resonance created to offer one of the most powerful healings that can happen."

This concept brought him back to his theory of dance as meditation. "In the world we live in, we are always worried about looking outside of us, trying to understand things and people around us. Being able to reach a meditative state is dependent on how well you are able to silence your mind and focus inward. When dancing blues with a partner, if you try to listen inwardly to the music as well as the inner flow of energy within yourself and your fellow partner, you may be able to experience this blissful state of mind, body and soul. It may be difficult for many people to let that happen initially because of how our minds have been conditioned to think, believe, judge, expect and react. However, I have found that blues does have the capacity to help us overcome that barrier and move toward bliss."

Krunal has experienced this healing himself, and he has witnessed it in his students. "People have told me they were healed in various ways after a blues dance— that the energy in their body was balanced out. It's not necessarily the dance itself. It is more about the connection that person had with the music and with their partner."

But Krunal was quick to say that, on a day-to-day basis, one can be in a state no longer requiring a dance partner in order to dance or in a state so that one can dance in order to appreciate music. "Blues dancing has taught me to be happy with myself even if there's nobody around me, just the music and myself. It has changed my life."

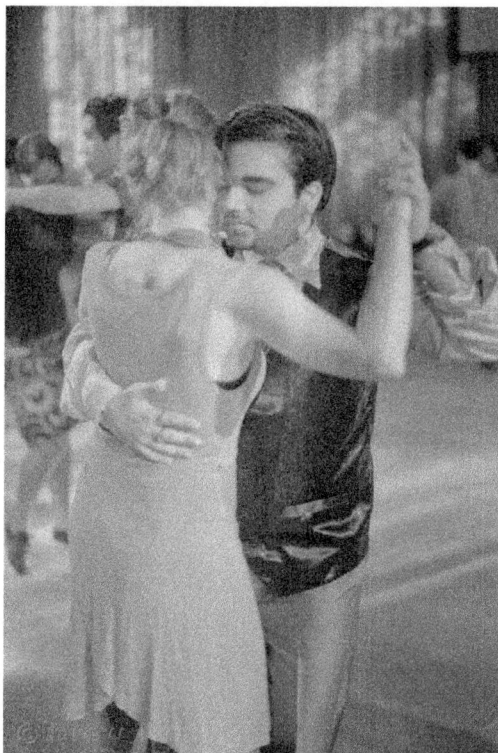
Photo by Drew Tronvig

A Dancer's Blessing

Stella, Portland, Oregon, USA

I first met Stella on a five-hour ride share to a Blues Recess dance event in northern Washington. Naturally, our conversation began with the topic of dancing, but it evolved into much deeper aspects of faith and inner conflict. I sat down with her for a formal interview the second day of the five-day event, for a recap of her journey through resolving the perceived paradox between God and blues dancing.

Stella shared that her family was part of an orthodox Presbyterian church on the East Coast until she was eight years old. "I started learning Latin in first grade; it was very much pointed in the direction of deeper biblical study." After her eighth birthday, her family moved to San Francisco, California, and continued with a Presbyterian church there. Although she had wanted to take dance classes as a child, she would not get the chance to indulge in her exploration of the arts until high school—when she was old enough to attend classes on her own.

The dance styles Stella participated in, such as tap and ballet, didn't exhibit much of a conflict with her spiritual beliefs—until she began blues dancing. The sexual undertones of the dance stood in deep contrast to what she'd been told was morally "right." She understood that "there's so much more to the blues than being sexy—like sorrow and tough times." But it was the "sexiness" that resulted in her inner conflict. "The issue was all the Christian dogma surrounding how you express, or I should say, how you do *not* express, your sexuality." Stella explained that, according to the teachings she'd been raised with, "outside of a certain place or time, it is inappropriate, rude, or even sinful to be a sexual being."

But once she started dancing, she couldn't stop that expression. "When I got on the dance floor and started loosening up, I couldn't stay stiff. It just came right out, and it felt so right and natural. And I got attention; I was acknowledged as someone who could dance and who was beautiful, and people wanted to dance with me. As a kid who wasn't popular, that was really seductive."

Stella left San Francisco soon after her discovery of the blues to attend college in Eugene, Oregon. Once settled in her new town, she immediately went about looking for places to blues dance. She found a growing blues dance community in Eugene, but it wasn't until she began traveling to Portland to attend dances that she started getting really immersed in the scene. "The blues dance floor was one place where I could express sensuality with it only *slightly* conflicting with my spiritual beliefs and convictions. I could make excuses for that conflict, because I wasn't actually *doing* anything. I was just shaking my hips on the dance floor, like I did in other dance styles."

Stella's immersion in the dance scene led to the development of what she considered opposing passions—which seemed to be reinforced among her social circles. "When I finally graduated college and stepped out into the world, I was really burned out. I'd had a ministry job at a church while I was finishing school and all of this volunteer work. What time remained to give to my social life was primarily within a Christian setting. When I left that world and I stopped going to church for the first time in twenty-three years, I was afraid that if I started talking about my spirituality and my religion in the blues scene in Portland, specifically—I'd been well-informed that Portland is one of the most un-churched cities in the US—that people would be hostile toward me. Then when it came to sharing my dance life with my friends from the church, I was again afraid of being judged. So for a long time I didn't share the other part of my life with either circle.

"I had these two different worlds; there were aspects of what I was doing on the dance floor that were borderline taboo in the Christian world. So these two passions were constantly in conflict, and I was stuck in the middle. It hurt. It was not a comfortable place to be."

Things began to change when Stella attended her first Blues Recess event, only a few months prior to our interview. Stella drove into the venue's parking lot, and the first order of business was to "take care of business." She found the nearest bathroom, sat down, and looked up. At eye level was a Bible verse on the bathroom stall door. "I just started laughing because this was Blues Recess—there's alcohol, there's lewd behavior, all sorts of activity that no respectful young Christian woman would ever expose herself to—and lo and behold it's being held in a retreat center that's founded and built for Mennonites. Here I was, in the middle of a Christian retreat campsite, about to embark on a weekend of God knows what, and I just started laughing."

Stella began a self-guided tour of the property, taking in all the pictures explaining the history of the site and the images of God. It was then that an overwhelming feeling of acceptance came over her. "Rather than feeling judged, rather than feeling like God was saying, 'You be careful now. I am watching you, and you better not do anything I've told you not to do,' what I heard were the words 'Even here I am with you. I am trusting you to do only what you're comfortable with. I love you. Carry on.' That was probably the highlight of the weekend—that sudden meshing of my two passions in my head and in my heart where I felt God accepting me and with me here."

Since then, Stella has established that her dancing is morally "right" for her. She concluded that it wasn't so much *what* she was doing on the dance floor that mattered—it was *why* she was doing it. "The conflict that happens now is less about the sexual aspect of dance conflicting with my religious practices and more about the question 'Is blues dancing something that you're doing because it brings you joy, or is it something that you're doing to get attention?' Fame and glory are not good reasons to dance, in my opinion. So that's where the conflict happens now. Occasionally I'll take a break from dancing for a little while and reevaluate my motives, but I always come back, get on the dance floor, and the biggest grin comes out on my face. The greatest compliment I can get is someone coming up to me and saying, 'I love to watch you dance. It brings me joy.'"

Stella has made great strides in her personal journey, but her experience at the second Blues Recess event, which we were at, made it clear she still had some work to do. "The challenge of this retreat isn't whether or not I should dance a certain way—it's figuring out the way I wish to behave when I'm not on the dance floor. And that's very complex, because there are so many contexts and relationships off the dance floor, and my desire is to be myself the whole way through."

This conflict became physical for Stella. "As soon as I arrived here, my anxiety manifested into this massively uncomfortable stomach ache. The pain was so uncomfortable. Obviously, this environment was creating a lot of stress for me. When my body is revolting on me so badly there's an instinct in me to figure out why—what's the cause of it and what am I so scared of?"

Thankfully, Stella had found members of the community she felt safe processing her feelings with, and she was able to discover the source of her pain and anxiety. "It is the duality of what's in my head. One side is a conditioned, judgmental reaction to what's going on around me, and the other side is so excited to not be forced to live a certain way based on rules that I didn't make for myself, that I haven't examined closely and accepted as my own."

It wasn't only what was going on around her that fed that duality, but also Stella's own actions. "The freer side of me is behaving in ways that I think are good for me and how I want to act, and then the judgmental side is judging me. It's a vicious circle, but I've been able to see how everything here has been affecting me and figure out ways to be kinder to myself, and in that process be kinder to the people around me."

It's not only at Blues Recess events that Stella explores how dancing fits into her life. "Blues dancing has become a huge part of my regular day to day life. I dance at the stop sign, I dance on the bus, I dance at work. If there's a beat somewhere I'm going to be moving to it. I'm not going to start booty shaking in the office, but dancing is everywhere in my life."

It is not only an outlet for self-expression that Stella has gained from dancing. Despite her initial hesitation to express her beliefs to the people she met outside her spiritual world, once she did, she was met with a surprising result. "If you're a part of the blues community, it generally means that there exists in you at least the desire for openness and transparency. That's not a rule, but it tends to be the case, so there are always good conversations to be had with blues dancers. The dance floor is the place where I can get dramatic and sassy and sexy and sad, and I can ask for comfort from somebody whom I've only known for three minutes."

As for her spiritual community, the reaction she got there surprised her too.

"When I did start sharing my dance world with some of my closest friends from my spiritual world, instead of them telling me I shouldn't be doing what I did and quoting Bible verses, they just listened. All they were interested in was that I was happy and that my experiences were what they needed to be for me.

"The friends I love and who love me are not here because they think I'm a good dancer, nor are they here because I walk the line of straight and narrow, nor because I'm the best at being Christian. They're here because they want to be with *me*." Which brought Stella back to her current challenge—and what I would call her triumph: "That's who I want to be, is me. The same me at all different levels, on or off the dance floor."

In the loft above the dance studio where we sat before the evening's organized activities commenced, Stella's attire led me to believe she had succeeded. She was adorning a scarf that she had fashioned into a dress. She was clearly not trying to be anyone else but herself. Stella may have heard God say it first, but she now repeats the same sentiment to herself as well: "I love you. Carry on."

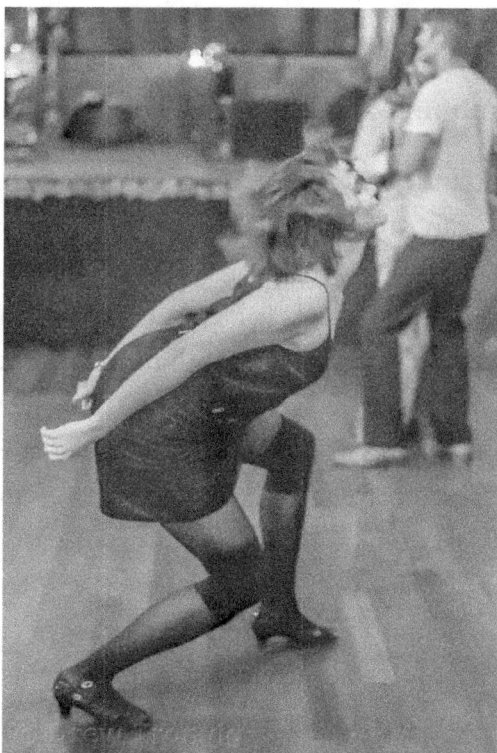

Photo by Drew Tronvig

The Tao of Dance

Surahbhi McMellahn, Devon, England

Surahbhi and her story came into my awareness as a result of an online post I'd written, asking if anyone could speak to the correlation between dance and Tao. Social media has a knack for connecting strangers with record speed. Later that day, Surahbhi reached out to tell me that dance was instrumental to her spiritual practice while living in an ashram. Her message stated:

"I spent from ages sixteen to thirty living with an enlightened master in India. Tao was one of the paths that he taught, and one that was very close to his heart and way of being." She shared that freestyle dance was one of the tools he used to practice this spiritual concept, "Dance was my meditation, and I explored it to the depths. Now, at fifty-five, I have discovered partner dancing and the blues, and I am drunk on it!"

Surahbhi's blues journey—like her life journey—has been all about the Taoist concept of "allowing." In other words, letting go. "When I dance, I am dissolving, letting go, allowing the music to completely move me without any ideas or interference. But at the same time, I need to be aware of the room, the music, the other dancers, and my dance partner—remaining disciplined and present. In the midst of the dissolution is integration. The dance disappears into the dancer; the dancer disappears into the dance. Who knows where I end and the other begins?"

Surahbhi spoke in a language that might sound foreign to those who haven't pursued a similar spiritual path. This path was foreign to her as well, upon her arrival in India from the United Kingdom. Dance, however, was not. "I was already into classical dance and wanted to train in dance, but when I got to India, it was very clear to me that my path was going to be an inner journey—not one of becoming a professional dancer."

However, the two worlds blended during her time at the ashram. "My teacher often spoke about how dance is one of the easiest and most natural paths inward—everyone can move, everyone responds to music, so it's the easiest technique to bring you within. You just close your eyes and begin moving your body." As Surahbhi would say, however, you have to first learn how to get out of your own way. "I had to unwind the human tendency to be the creator, to not let fear get in the way and just let go and be taken over by the music. I had to learn how to not be there—not be a rock in the water but just let the water flow."

After she returned to the United Kingdom, dance would not reenter her life for many years. Music entered it first. She fell in love with a blues and Celtic guitarist. "We started writing Celtic folk songs together, and I began singing. A singing teacher had showed me a technique where you strengthen your diaphragm, which is the third chakra, representing power and expansion into the world. I could feel this was really doing the right thing for me, making me feel like I'm here, and I have a voice."

Although the romantic relationship would end after seven years, the two would continue singing and performing together for another fifteen years before he fell ill and their career paths separated. As she sang and performed less, space was made in her life to explore other creative outlets. She felt it was time to try out dancing again. She began dancing modern jive, which led her to discover blues dancing. "When I first started, it was just with a few steps in close embrace. At the end of the song, I said, 'Oh my god, what happened?' Suddenly there was this synchronicity of our two bodies, and I didn't know if he was leading me or if I did that. I turned to my partner with my mouth gaped open and said, 'I didn't know where you ended and I began.' I really didn't. I was just letting it happen."

From that first blues dance, Surahbhi felt a new world open up to her—one of which she kept coming back to for more. "There's something magical for me about partner dancing. I never got those heightened experiences dancing alone. I could feel them wanting to happen, but somehow there was something missing. Dancing the blues has been like the missing part of a jigsaw puzzle. It has shown me that something more can happen. I don't know whether it's the male-female polarity, but it doesn't happen for me without that presence."

She also found, to her surprise, that she fell in love with the music. "I started really listening to blues music for the first time. My partner had always raved about blues. As a musician I didn't like it at first, because it's incredibly basic—I liked the more mysterious stuff." As it turned out, she simply hadn't yet found the artists she resonated with. "I started to discover these amazing musicians—Robert Cray, B. B. King, Eric Clapton, Joe Bonamassa."

Surahbhi had remained close friends with her former life and music partner, and she shared with him her discovery, "I told him 'Ohmigosh! I just discovered this incredible song!' I played him 'The Bluest Blue,' by Alvin Lee, and he just laughed and said, 'That's probably the most famous blues song ever,' and here I was hearing it for the first time. And I was just totally in love with it. It was beautiful."

At about this time, her friend's health—he'd been diagnosed with pancreatic cancer—had deteriorated to the point where he could no longer play music at all. However, the two began enjoying music together in a different way. "We'd go camping and lie on our backs by the sea, and we'd listen to these blues tracks. To fall in love with the rawness in the electric guitar being played, and to feel the raw suffering of this man beside me...it was like I was saying good-bye to one beloved and hello to another."

Surahbhi would lose both her beloved and her mother around the same time. It was their passing that led to a revelation for her: "Love is nothing like what I'd been thinking it was. Just for a moment I saw what it is: it's *huge*. It's way beyond our small worries and concerns." With this understanding, she found a coping mechanism for her pain. "Through the blues, I could dance my grief and loss so totally and passionately until it burned through to a love and joy so much bigger than myself and my own personal losses.

"Pain and loss are there, that's part of being a human being. But I found that if I kept dancing and just kept allowing the pain to flow through me, not holding a little back because it was too frightening to go all the way, if I just allowed it to do what it wanted to do, it would always come through to love." Surahbhi, once again, lost track of where one ended and the other began.

"I danced until love was dancing me. When I step onto the dance floor, I intend to empty myself, and Tao is the vessel I use for that. I try and be empty. That's how I dance my way to love—I release everything that's in me until I'm empty. I find that place where there is no Surahbhi there—her ideas, her desires or expectations, her choices, her opinions. Just what is. I surrender to the music, to my partner, to what is. That, to me, is the Tao of blues dancing."

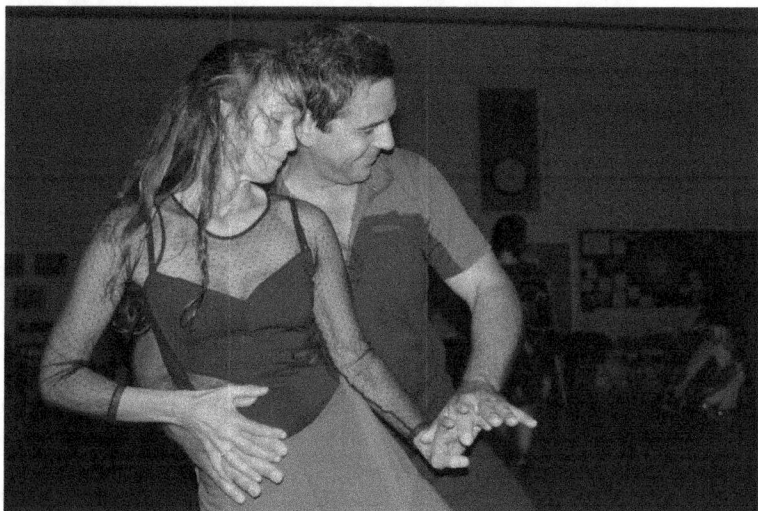

A Soul Kind of Girl

Liraz Shveka, Rishon Lezion, Israel

Liraz's story was difficult to categorize for this book, because her blues journey is all-encompassing of the body-mind-soul triad. Each aspect of her well-being has been equally influenced by dance. However, I am including her story in this section because in my opinion, transformations of the body and mind begin with the soul.

Interestingly enough, Liraz's introduction to dancing of any kind was not through a class or a social event. It was through Xbox. Three years ago, her sister bought the video device, which came with a game called *Dance Central*. The system's camera could see you and read your body movements; your job was to imitate the dance movements made on screen. She considered the game a good source of exercise and found that she could imitate the dance moves quite naturally.

Dancing freestyle in her room was one thing, but she still was resistant and uncomfortable with the idea of going to a wedding or party and dancing in public. She continued with her "private" dance parties for a while, until one of her colleagues at the school where she is a music teacher invited her to a swing band event.

She accepted the invitation and had an unexpected experience—she became enthralled by a group of dancers at the event. "I'd never seen anyone dancing like that in Israel, or even in the world. I didn't know swing dancing existed." She went home that night and searched online for places to learn in Tel Aviv. She found one that had a weekly beginner's course starting ten days later. "That was enough time to let it sink in but not too long to make me change my mind." Liraz grinned at her reasoning. She attended the first class and had a positive experience. "The music was really nice—it's the music that moves me; I love swing music. And the atmosphere was really warm. So I thought, okay, I'm willing to commit for one month."

The course was an enjoyable experience for her, but she wasn't yet hooked. "It was nice, but everybody told me I'd get addicted, and I didn't see how that could happen to me. Everyone was a beginner, so there were people dancing with no feel for the rhythm, and being a music teacher, I have a very difficult time following someone who is not following the beat. But I kept on going, and I realized later that the four to five hours a week that I was in class, I didn't think about work." Liraz had become consumed by her job. She wasn't even sure she wanted to continue being a music teacher. She found dancing to be a healthy escape mechanism from her mind, at least that one night per week. "Dancing was what allowed me to escape being on the verge of real depression. Dance rescued me," she divulged.

After three or four months taking classes, Liraz began to understand what everyone meant by the dance being addictive. She would finish a class and her thoughts would instantly go to, "Where is the next class?

Where is the next class?" Liraz laughed now at her state of mental urgency.

The school also offered balboa and blues classes. "I didn't go to blues at first. I felt it was too close, too intimate. But after a while I tried balboa. Balboa was okay—it was intimate, but not like blues dancing. In balboa, you connect with your chest and shoulders only, not your pelvis. 'Blues dancing is for dirty people,' I thought." She laughed again at her logic.

Liraz came to realize that what she liked most about balboa was, in fact, the intimacy. Dancing balboa felt like a hug. "After my day at work, I'd want someone to give me a hug. I'd look at the calendar and go, 'Okay, there's a Lindy Hop class tonight—that's nice. But afterward is balboa. Yay, balboa! I get to sleep in somebody's arms!' That's what it felt like. It's very calming and soothing."

Then, about a year ago, she felt like she could try blues. "I went to London last summer, and one of my swing teachers said, 'Whatever you do, just go for a blues class with Vicci and Adamo. Even if you don't like blues dancing, just go to a class with them—you'll enjoy yourself.' So I went, and she was right. They were so charming and amazing, and the class was so nice—the atmosphere, the pub, everything." Liraz returned to Tel Aviv enthusiastic about trying blues dancing.

"I wouldn't have been able to start blues dancing without Lindy Hop and balboa first. Those dances made me feel comfortable in somebody's arms. I needed stages to get to the level of intimacy with blues dancing." Liraz began taking blues dance classes, and found the scene very welcoming and not judgmental. "Blues is very accepting. You just have to be a musical person, a good spirit, and a kind soul to be a dancer that people want to dance with."

With blues added to her repertoire, Liraz found herself out dancing nearly every night of the week. "I had the blues class on Sunday; then Monday if I had the strength and energy, I would go to a Lindy Hop party hosted by another school; Tuesday I had balboa and Lindy Hop classes; Wednesday there was nothing"— Liraz groaned to emphasize her disappointment in that fact—"Thursday was the Lindy Hop party at my school; Friday there were street parties; and Saturday night another Lindy Hop party. It's a full week of dancing. When I'm on holidays, I dance every single night of the week."

Dancing became more than a distraction for Liraz and more than a form of physical exercise. It became nearly her entire social life. "I see my dance friends twice a week on school nights, every day on holidays. My non-dance friends I don't see as often. Sometimes I have to remind myself that I have a life outside of dance—that I have good non-dance friends I should give some attention to as well. And that sometimes I can do things outside of dancing and still enjoy myself." I noticed a glint in her eye.

As a music teacher, she finds that music is the most important element when she's deciding to dance or not. It helped, therefore, that blues music moves her.

"I *love* the music. It's really…*grrrrrrr.*" Liraz made a guttural sound, emphasizing how deeply within her body that feeling goes. "I'm a soul kind of girl. When the music goes into that soul direction, *that* is my territory. My *ahhhh,* oh my *god* territory."

Aside from the music, the other element that brings Liraz to that heightened state is the intimacy with her dance partner. "The best dances I have include a combination of songs that I like and a very high level of intimacy with someone I feel comfortable with. Intimacy is not something to be taken lightly. Intimacy is not sex. At first I thought blues dancing was something I would only do as long as I don't have a boyfriend, but recently I've been thinking, there's no reason to give it up. I enjoy leading girls as well; yes, there's probably something more when I dance with a guy—there's always that extra tension—but the intimacy is there even when I dance with a girl. Maybe we're missing intimacy in this life; maybe we should give it more space and opportunity to let it grow and flourish."

Liraz has learned that intimacy doesn't have to be between two people who know each other, either. "I've learned that I can create intimacy with many people and feel comfortable with it. Even with complete strangers, it can be so deep that the music ends, and you're still dizzy from the feeling of connection; it's so obvious to both of you that you can't destroy the moment—you have to keep on dancing. It's too soon to end it."

So much of her time is devoted to dance that Liraz can't remember what her life was like before dancing. "What was I doing with all that time? I didn't have any hobbies before. Dancing is the first thing in my life that is not an idle activity, like watching TV or eating or doing something that is not good for you. Ice cream was always my favorite thing in life. The other day, I was taking a nap in the afternoon and I hardly managed to wake up, but I woke up because I had a Lindy class and party. I was thinking to myself, 'I wouldn't get up now even to eat ice cream. But I *am* getting up to dance. Do I like dancing more than I like ice cream?'"

Since swing and blues dancing had been unheard of by Liraz, I wondered how her friends perceived her dancing—and also the Tel Avivian society in general. As Liraz identifies as an atheist, there was no religious conflict for her with the dance, although there is still resistance to the intimacy of blues dancing in her culture. "There's no problem in the culture here with partner dancing in general, it's not perceived as something dirty. I think people perceive Lindy Hop as cool when they see it; it's very innocent and playful and nonsexual, so it's very easy to digest, even for those outside the city. You don't need to be a liberal Tel Avivi to accept Lindy Hop. Even my fellow teachers, my boss, they know about my Lindy Hop dancing. I've shown them clips, and they think it looks fun. It's not something that's taboo. But I wouldn't show them blues dancing.

"I think for most outsiders it's very difficult to understand. You have to try it in order to understand it. Otherwise it looks outside of your world, like, 'That's for *those* people,' but I think you just have to try it to understand what it means and what it does to your body, to your mind, to your soul.

"It's understandable that it's difficult for people to accept blues dancing. It's difficult for people to see intimacy. If you go down the street and you see people kissing, will you keep on looking? Probably not. I think it embarrasses people to watch intimacy. So perhaps it's very embarrassing for some people to watch blues dancing. You have to know that this intimacy is a very certain kind of intimacy before you realize it's okay to watch it."

I asked Liraz what role she saw culture or religion playing in the acceptance of displays of intimacy. "As a society, I don't think Israel is more conservative or religious than American society—maybe even less, and especially Tel Aviv. Tel Aviv is very liberal, so I don't think religion has anything to do with the perception of partner dancing. It is just a society thing. Just like in the States, it doesn't suit everyone to meet strangers and offer them a dance. There are many barriers that people have to cross in order to start dancing, or watch dancing, or love dancing."

Perhaps, like Liraz, they could start with Xbox. You never know where a good game of *Dance Central* might lead.

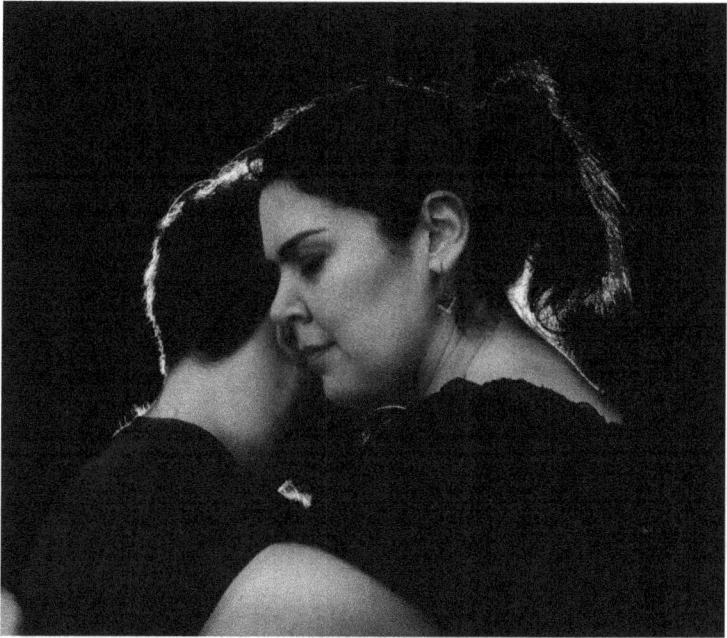

Photo by Alexandre Swidaneel

V
SOCIAL

The stories in this section carry a central theme around social relationships—life lessons learned through dance about friendships or romantic relationships; the discovery of a world in which social environments doesn't cause anxiety; the enrichment of life due to opportunities to engage with those from different generations, professional fields, or cultures…The list goes on.

For some, the dance community was the first community they ever felt a part of at all. Ellie Westgarth, from London, England, shared, "The blues community helped me feel at home in my own city. In the modern world, especially in a city as large as London, people can be quite disconnected. What blues has taught me to do is treat everyone I meet as a friend straight away."

The transformation such a shift can elicit has no bounds. One of the greatest pleasures I had while interviewing people for this book was witnessing a somewhat bashful personality blossom into one whose words flowed with ease and boundless joy. All it took was asking them to tell me about their passion. When we locate that inner spark, it can be massaged into a raging fire.

Not everyone in this section needed encouragement—some merely required a quiet listener. The beauty of the human spirit was revealed either way: we are creatures of connection. Social engagement—

whether it comes naturally or with great effort—is important to our well-being. Here are six stories of social lives transformed through blues dancing.

Learning to Like Having Friends

Devon Cooke, Vancouver, BC, Canada

When Devon began telling me his blues story, it first appeared to be about the body. However, as he continued, it became clear it was about how he *uses* the body in order to access the parts of himself that allow him to open his heart to others. His journey of transformation from a self-described "workaholic loner" to someone who "finally understands why people want to interact with each other" began at an alternative blues—or fusion—dance exchange in 2010. It was the first time he'd immersed himself in dance for an entire weekend, and he described the experience as "revelatory."

"I'd never really spent a significant amount of time paying attention to my body before that event. It opened my eyes to a world that I had basically ignored." Although the whole event was transformational for him, one particular class stands out in Devon's memory. It was an African dance class on body mechanics, taught by a man born and raised in Africa.

"It was a Saturday morning. I had already done a full day of classes and danced all night. I was breaking in new dance shoes, and my body hurt—my back was locked up; my shins were like stones; I couldn't step. I could barely straighten up."

What made this class so different from any other class Devon had taken was that the teacher wasn't after having the students move their bodies in a certain way—he was after having them open up their hearts. He had the students take off their shoes and follow his lead as he stomped on the ground with great effort.

"He would point out when we were getting tired, when we weren't giving our all and throwing our hearts into it fully. It was pretty intense, a serious workout. I was exhausted, and my body was sore—I had a million reasons to not give it my all. But he was really good at getting that heart out of me, so I threw myself into it."

The revelation Devon spoke of was that by the end of the class, all of the stiffness and soreness his body carried at the start of class had disappeared. "My body was fine for the rest of the weekend. I really needed to go into that intense physical space to realize that that level of intensity could heal."

After that, Devon started paying attention to the subtleties of his body's messages. After each class he would ask himself, "What felt good? What didn't feel good? What movement was possible, what wasn't possible? Where am I sensitive and why?" Answering these questions would bring him significant insight into his mind—and his heart.

"I learned how to be in my body and what that does for me as a person. This wasn't just paying attention to my body, it was paying attention *with* my body. It was moving my center of consciousness from my brain into my gut, so I could experience my physical existence directly and viscerally."

The disappearance of his sore muscles was the

most immediate effect of being in his body, but he'd come to realize that the effects were much more far reaching. "When I'm in my body, I'm more confident, I'm nicer, I'm more sociable, and I'm more sensitive. I make better judgments. I am happier, more generous, and more loving. I experience the world more fully and can offer more of myself in return."

As a result, Devon began to gain the courage to reach out to others and to appreciate being part of a community. "I was an introvert and a loner for most of my life. I'd never been to an event where I felt so totally accepted by a community. I don't think I ever really understood what it meant to be part of a community.

"But at the dance event, I made the connection that when I was in my body, I wasn't worrying about what other people were thinking or what to say. I was able to stop my brain from telling me these stories about how I was bad at social interaction or how someone didn't like me."

Encompassed in Devon's fear of social interaction was the fear of sexual interaction. Dancing helped him there too. "It gave me a social construct where I was comfortable enough to talk to women, be attracted to women, and not have that whole fear around having to act on it."

He believed his fear around expressing his masculinity and sexuality began in grade school as a result of circumstances when he was bullied, but he felt the same message emphasized by modern culture and media as he came into adulthood. "I feel men are portrayed as aggressors in our society. To a certain extent we demonize our sexualities, so I had a pretty significant fear of my own sexuality. Eventually I did learn how to be comfortable with my sexuality and to express attraction, and that has changed the way that I approach relationships. I'm still on that journey. I'm a lot more accepting of myself than I was, and dance definitely has been a big part of that.

"I've also become aware of how important human touch is to general health and how much that is missing for so many people. Dancing is an environment where it's normal to hug people. When I go back into the rest of the world—and particularly in a business networking environment—I have to remind myself it's not normal to hug someone after you've said hi."

Devon is actually in the midst of attempting to make his business world and his dance world intermingle. He operates his own video production company, which specializes in making corporate videos. However, he realized his filmmaking skills could be useful in promoting dance. He has since worked to create videos for the swing, fusion, and blues dance communities.

He does what he can to expose others to the healing power of dance, which includes making new community members feel as welcome as he was made to feel. Dancers who have been around the scene for a while tend to stick to their "favorite" follows or leads, but Devon has recognized that a new favorite could be a brand-new member to the scene. "A lot of my favorite moments are dancing with first-time dancers. I love making a connection with someone who is just giving me their experience raw, not through lessons or skills or any of that. I think dancing can sometimes take us out of touch with ourselves for the sake of technique. When I meet a first-time dancer who just has instincts—the only skills she has are those instincts—and if I can get in touch with my own instincts and those play together, there's a lot of discovery that happens. Some of my best dances come out of that."

Spoken like a man who is not afraid of intimacy. It made me wonder what would happen if all of humanity took a class like the African dance one that he took—if we were all led to "throw down" until our hearts opened fully.

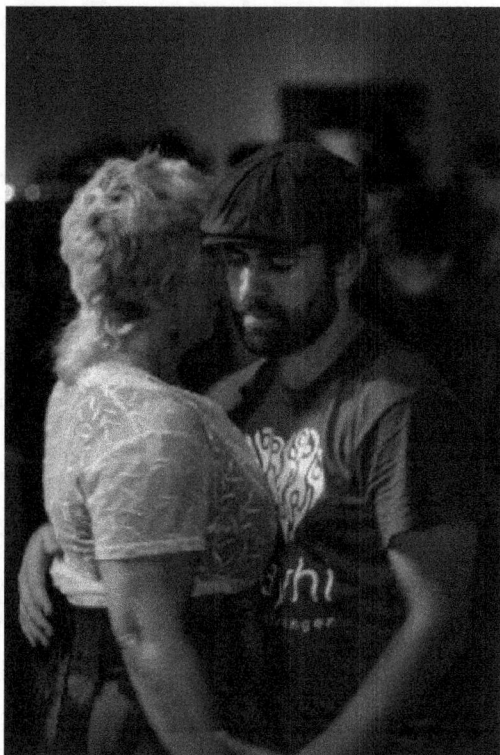

Photo by Alexey Tolstoguzov

This Is What It Means to Be Human

Leonard Krause, Eugene, Oregon, USA

Most people I've met on the blues dance floor come there having had either no dance experience or some experience with another partnered social dance. If you have just one dance with Leonard, or even watch him dance for a few moments, you'll notice his background is different. Leonard was professionally trained in numerous styles of dance and movement—starting with ballet.

Leonard and I sat on a couch in his makeshift "living room" at a Blues Recess event while he told me his story. Most attendees at the event simply had brought a small tent, but the arrangement Leonard's roommate constructed truly was remarkable. A canopy hung over a temporary home—a full-size bed, kitchen, and the space in which we sat. Curtains hung between each "room," various carpets were laid out, and lights hung around the perimeter. Leonard offered me a cup of tea before we settled onto the couch, which overflowed with colorful pillows.

As I'd soon discover, however, Leonard doesn't "settle" for long. Repeatedly he felt a memory or a term required demonstration for further emphasis, and he bolted onto his feet, striking a ballet or samurai pose, for example. None of this surprised me after I learned about his background in mime—but ballet came first.

"The first ballet class I took was when I was sixteen or seventeen years old, and if you're a guy, there are two main challenges to that. The first is walking upstairs to the ballet studio and saying, 'I'm here for the lesson.'" Leonard lowered his gaze and made himself smaller, remembering what it felt like all these years later. "The second is I had to buy a dance belt and tights." A dance belt is similar to a thong, used to support male ballet dancers' most sensitive region. Leonard was determined to make it through those two challenges, however, due to his long-held desire to dance.

"I fell in love with ballet when I was ten years old. My parents took me to see *Swan Lake*, and what I recall is how the dancers had such amazing control over their bodies. It impressed me so much." Leonard filed that memory away, along with another from when he was twelve years old.

"I used to stay up late and watch Johnny Carson's show. One night Marcel Marceau—the mime—was on. I thought it was the most incredible thing, to use your body to tell a story. Something with that resonated with me."

Then, while he was attending what he describes as a "hippie high school" in Washington, DC, a woman who had danced with the Martha Graham Dance Company was brought to his school to teach a modern dance class. He became so enthralled with dance performance that a friend suggested he study dance. "It was one of those defining moments when I realized,

229

'Wow, you can study dance in college?' Everything came together then: my need to entertain people, my love of movement, and the discipline I had that would allow me to train professionally."

He didn't waste any time getting started. In addition to enrolling in ballet class, he registered for a summer course at American University and began studying modern dance with the Eric Hawkins Dance Company—run by the former husband of Martha Graham. However, his start there wasn't so smooth. "I was kicked out of his repertory class because I loved ballet too much—he was anti-ballet. The only other choice for that time slot was pantomime. So, instead, I started studying mime."

Although he continued to study dance while attending Middlebury College in Vermont—averaging two hours per day in the dance studio all four years—his major was in Spanish. While studying in Spain during his junior year of college, it was his mime skills that allowed him to make a living. "I used to average twenty dollars per hour as a street performer. In today's dollars, that's over seventy per hour."

Just when I thought Leonard's story could not have gotten any more diverse, he began to tell me about the period when he lived in Japan.

"During my senior year of college, I applied for and received a fellowship to study traditional theater in Japan—mostly due to my previous study in dance and physical theater. I was there from September of 1979 to March of 1983. During that time, I studied Kyogen (the traditional comedy performed during acts of Noh plays) and Kabuki from Nakamura Matazo, from the National Theatre. The grant lasted for only one year, so I had to find other sources of income. I worked as an English teacher, a dancer and physical theater performer, a TV and movie actor, and for a small trading company. The trading company sent me to the States to run an oil exploration company based in Medford, Oregon…which is how I met my wife."

I had to take a deep breath to allow the plethora of experiences that had made up Leonard's rich life to sink in. The idea that so much can lie behind a dance partner's face and embrace that most often goes unmentioned was emphasized as our talk continued.

"Alison was one of the first people I met when I came back to the States in 1984. We met on Valentine's Day. She had an office in the same suite as mine. We married in 1987. She had a five-year-old son from her previous marriage, so I was an instant father. I used to dance by myself to stay in shape, but at the time, the opportunity for partner dancing was limited. It would be another ten years before I started partner dancing again.

"We lived down the street from the Tango Center in Eugene, Oregon, and Alison suggested that we dance tango for New Year's, which we did. She still had problems moving due to complications from an operation she had years before, so she did not really get into it. I, on the other hand, found my love of dance rekindled. I totally went for it."

Leonard began attending dance events around the region, including a tango festival in Seattle, where he had a life-transforming experience as a result of one particular teacher.

"There was a teacher there named Tete Rusconi. He was in his seventies. Tete had the incredible ability to be able to dance with anybody. I was in an advanced class with him, and we were short one follow. So he says to somebody in class, 'Go out and find a woman—just any woman walking down the hall.' So the person goes out and comes back with a woman that probably weighed about 280 pounds, who had just started dancing tango. Every time I tell this story, it almost makes me cry. Tete took her hand, walked her into the center, held her in an embrace, did the move, stepped back, and said, 'This is how it's done.' He had so much love, so much generosity of heart, and so much respect for the people he danced with. I asked him to lead me, to show me one move, and even then, it was like, oh my god." Leonard paused momentarily as tears brimmed in his eyes. "There was so much love in that one moment."

Leonard's takeaway from that experience is one that he has carried with him each dance since then. "He taught me that the essence of what dance is, is love. Behind your dance partner is a soul, a human being who has feelings, who has problems. Every partner I dance with, there's only ever been one. And we may never see each other again, so I ask myself, 'Can I make this moment together ultimate love, ultimate respect?' It's at that moment where I feel, oh my god," Leonard didn't try to hold back his tears. "This is what it's like to be a human being. To be able to honor Tete, I try to take that philosophy of generosity of heart into every dance."

By this point in the interview, I had become enthralled by Leonard's authenticity. I hadn't known what to expect of his story—we'd met only briefly the night before, when we'd shared an enchanting dance. I should not have been surprised, therefore, by his exhibition of such raw emotion. It did not make me uncomfortable; in fact, nothing could have pleased me more. I was discovering a kindred spirit. He soon shared, however, that he hadn't always been so in touch with his own humanity or so appreciative of the humanity of others.

After having trained in professional dance performance since the age of sixteen, he found that partner dancing required a reframing of how he saw himself in relationship to other dancers. "When you're a trained dancer, your partners are kind of like performance objects. Not that you don't relate to them as human beings, but you're more concerned with how the dance looks as a function. As a performance artist, you undergo physical training that becomes so ingrained in all aspects of your life; you spend so much time on how you look."

Leonard learned the hard way the adverse effect that kind of mindset can have on one's relationships. "When I think about my marriage...I pushed my wife through tango. For a certain period of time, I would push my dance partners because I felt that how they looked was a reflection of me. It's like, if you're a parent, you want your kids to look a certain way because they reflect you as a parent. I learned later that the appearance of others has nothing to do with me, but it was too late for my marriage."

At the time Leonard's marriage was coming to an end, a friend of his was working to develop a blues dance scene in Eugene. She invited him to a dance, and his initial reaction was, with a hint of sarcasm, "Blues dance, what the heck is *blues* dance?" She asked him to watch a video of the dance online, to which his reaction changed: "Oh my god, this is what we used to dance after ballet class when I was growing up!" Leonard described the pressure of having to execute perfect, symmetrical movements in ballet and how hours of this at a time led to his colleagues and him needing to release some of the physical tension.

"After dance class, somebody would crank up different music, and we'd let ourselves go. We needed to shake up our bodies and just *be* with each other."

He went with his friend to a local blues dance, and once again became engrossed in the freedom to dance in whatever style suited him. He immediately enjoyed an observation: "Everybody has what I call their native language. Their body moves in a certain way, depending on their culture, their parents and how they grew up, and just how their body responds to music. I have my own definite style—I'm the only one that flails his arms like a ballet dancer." Leonard laughed, without a hint of regret.

He also noticed that this new community of his was very generationally diverse. "Our society is so stratified by age. What in our society brings people of different ages together? There's really not much, but blues dance is one of the few things. What's amazing to me is there can be this sense of physical connectedness across generations that is just so life-affirming to me."

And not just physical connectedness by contact but by communication. "Just by dancing with you, I *get* you. And you get me. I think ultimately as human beings we really want to be seen. We want to be seen for who we are. And that's what blues dance has opened up for me."

Though the blues dance scene does span across multiple generations, there are still challenges that a middle-aged man such as Leonard has to overcome. "I remember the first time I came to a blues dance event. I mean, I'm balding, right? I look like a middle-aged guy. So there's always this moment when I ask a woman to dance—she'll be in her twenties—and I get this look. You'd have to be me to see it, but it's like, 'Oh my god...'" Leonard began breathing deeply, his eyes large. 'Oh no...my father's asking me to dance. Please god, no.'"

To be honest, I am probably guilty of having given Leonard that look the night before, albeit with a bit more subtlety. But as soon as the first beat of the song we danced to hit, any hesitation was overridden by absolute pleasure. Like in the interview, he wasn't afraid to wear his heart out on his sleeve, and I used that as an invitation to put mine out there too. Dancing with Leonard was an emotional experience but also a playful one. His ballet moves inspired me to add in my tango moves, and together we stretched the boundaries of experimentation. As Leonard described, dance is about "cocreation"—and not just with your partner but among your own body, mind, and spirit.

"When you allow yourself to fully cocreate, there's this transcendent moment when you *are* the dance. It's a moment that is not part of the time-space continuum. It allows us all to meet in a completely mutual environment.

"At a Blues Recess event like this one, we talk about this 'consent culture.' We didn't have this language when I was growing up—it just wasn't in the consciousness of society. I see dance as one continuum of consent. Dance is an invitation and an ascension. I invite you to do this, and you say yes or no. The way you say yes or no is just with your weight. If I invite you to come toward me and you do—and it can be so subtle—then you've said yes. If you hold your ground, you've said no, and we're left going in a different direction. In essence, for a dance to work, it has to be mutual."

Leonard went on to describe what happens in a dance that is not working. "If I'm dancing, and my partner is speaking her language, and I pull her off her center, it's like a conversation where somebody interrupts you. The conversation keeps going, but you get this feeling like, 'I'm not being heard.' However, when it's totally consensual, when it flows, that's the juice in life."

It goes back to the human desire to feel seen. "To be seen, we have to be vulnerable and authentic ourselves. And we have to feel safe in order to do that. You probably have some partners where you go, 'You know what—I'm not going to open up my heart. I don't trust this person enough to give of myself.' This is where I think dance can be transformative. If we understand the signals of people, I believe blues dance can make people better human beings."

Leonard spoke from experience. He has applied these concepts in his own life, off the dance floor. "This is an example of one of the ways that blues dance especially has transformed my life. As a performer and an insecure person, I used to feel like I had to entertain people and fill up empty space—that I always needed to be funny and charming. Those qualities kept me from opening up to other people—in my marriage and other relationships. They teach you in ballet that your job as a dance partner is to always anticipate and always be there; whereas in blues dance, there's a give and take. I realized through blues dancing that I needed to become a better listener. If you feel listened to as a dancer when I dance with you, I feel I was successful as a co-dancer."

Recalling our dance from the night before, I know that I not only felt listened to but also fully accepted. Leonard had mastered the art of nonverbal communication—and, I was discovering throughout the interview, verbal as well. He required little effort on my part for guidance—just as he danced from the heart, he spoke from the heart, and his words flowed in such a way that I dared not interrupt.

"Looking back on my life, the possibility that dance brings is that as human beings we don't like to feel uncomfortable. But unless we're willing to be in that place, there's really no access to anything else. It's like armoring. You can't move in armor. You have to be vulnerable to be authentic. Watching blues dancers, watching their unabashed physical intimacy, I kind of feel sad on one end, because it makes me think how there's a lot of physical intimacy—and I don't mean sexual intimacy—lacking in our culture.

"In Western culture, physical contact is either among family members or through a romantic partner. I think because of the way our culture has become— either you're this or you're that—we are not given permission to walk down the street arm and arm with our friends. We have all these terms here to define our behavior; we try to put these labels on things that describe a facet of humanity."

Leonard paused and took a deep breath, as though digging up a beloved memory. "While living in Japan, I was able to visit Tibet. I spent three weeks hanging out with monks at a monastery. And you know, this is going to make me cry, but we would just snuggle into each other; we'd be in contact. There's something so healing, so nurturing, and so bonding in that. I think it's a way for people to recharge their human batteries. And I think dance satisfies that urge people have to be bonded to somebody else. We've given it a title: 'nonsexual snuggling' or 'nonsexual contact.' But you know what? I call it being human."

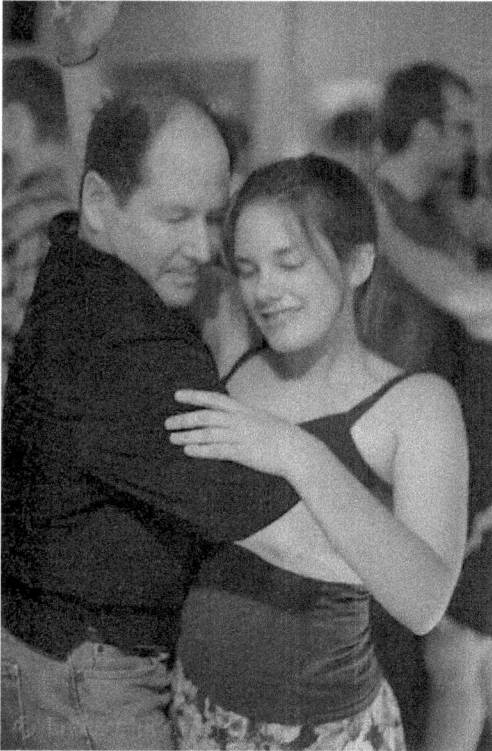

Photo by Drew Tronvig

Age Doesn't Matter

Jill Grant, Halifax, Nova Scotia, Canada

Most contributors to this book came to me through word of mouth. A few, however, responded to the call for stories I posted on my website. That post included several introductory questions I asked all potential contributors to answer, so that I could prepare a more tailored follow-up discussion. Jill was the only person who responded to my post who took the time to thoughtfully answer the questions before our interview. I was not surprised, therefore, when she shared that she's a university professor. Knowing what it's like to conduct research—and complete homework—she graciously made my job easier.

When we met through video conference for our interview, her countenance was professional and poised, and I could clearly picture her at the front of a classroom. Once she began speaking of her love of blues music and dance, however, her body relaxed, her voice softened, and her words took on a more natural flow. Soon, I would learn how blues dancing had helped soften her strictly academic world into one of late-night grooves, sensual moves, and a social circle that spanned all ages.

"I first got excited about blues music in the 1960s, when many of the early rock acts—like the Beatles, the Rolling Stones, Canned Heat, and Jimi Hendrix—were playing with blues music in new ways.

Growing up, we listened to Detroit radio—Motown, soul, and R&B were on the radio all the time."

What she loved about the music was that it made her want to dance. "I love the emotion and the complex rhythms of blues music. I can't stop myself from pulsing and wanting to dance when blues music comes on. I had learned about jive and jitterbug as a child, because my parents and babysitter were dancers. Dancing was something I grew up assuming everybody did."

Even so, she didn't study dance herself. "I remember asking my mother if I could take dance lessons while I was tap-dancing down the grocery store aisle when she was shopping, and she said, 'No, we can't afford it.' But now I can afford it, so I indulge myself in the opportunity."

Her journey to dancing began in 2005 when her daughter started swing dancing. She was so enthusiastic about it that Jill decided to try it for herself. At one point, a visiting instructor offered an hour lesson in blues. She observed others who felt the connection to blues music that she did and who were confident interpreting the music creatively with their bodies. Despite feeling a significant age difference between herself and the other dancers, she felt "welcomed and appreciated."

She knew she wanted to explore this new community further, but it would take several years. In 2011, Jill decided to "take the plunge" and drove with two friends the twelve-hour journey from Halifax, Nova Scotia, to Boston, Massachusetts, for a blues weekend workshop. "It was a chance to start learning some real techniques, since we didn't have instructors here in Halifax." Since then, Jill has tried to attend several blues dance workshops a year, even though it involves traveling a great distance. "When I go, I take advantage of the opportunity for private lessons with top-notch instructors. In that way, I've been able to improve my dancing and get to the point where I can help others learn how to blues dance."

Jill has since become one of the more experienced dancers in her community and generously offers up what she has learned—in the realm of both teaching and deejaying blues dances—so she may share with others what she has come to love. "I enjoy teaching. It forces me to break down what's going on in the moves and think about what it takes for someone else to work on technique and become a better dancer. I get a lot of satisfaction from other people feeling like they're developing their own abilities and becoming more comfortable with the dance."

Of course, teaching in general is nothing new for Jill. However, the blues classroom is quite different from the academic university classroom. "I tend to step into an adult-figure role, for two reasons. I do travel a lot, so I have a growing amount of experience that I can share with people. But I also probably get seen as a more senior dancer in the scene not just in terms of experience but because of an age element too. I'm the oldest dancer—I'm old enough to be the grandmother of some of the kids I'm dancing with. As a university professor, I'm always around young people, so that's nothing new to me, but I don't generally socialize with students except in work-related events. Because of dancing, I get invited to all kinds of things that I would never have gotten invited to. I don't always go, but dance creates these social connections so that young people don't think of me necessarily as an old lady first, but as a dancer first. Dancing has been a good way for me to make different kinds of friendships—with people of different backgrounds, ages, education, and interests."

Jill described herself as an introvert who is in many ways "not so keen on socializing." However, she has found through blues dancing that she loves to connect with others in a nonverbal way. "I enjoy the physicality of partner dancing. I like the challenge of working with a partner to make something that feels beautiful."

The effects of her experience on the dance floor have transferred over to her life as a professor. "Blues dancing has had a profound influence on my life. Before I got into it, I spent almost all my time on my work—sixty to eighty hours a week working on course preparation, grading, research, and writing. Since I got into blues dancing and deejaying, I save time for listening to music, planning sets, planning dance lessons, and dancing whenever I can. Now I plan blues dance travel into my schedule and work around it. Blues has given me a creative outlet that uses different parts of my brain and body than my daily life and work do."

The transition wasn't a natural one for her, however. She had to overcome the belief that the people in her professional life shouldn't know about her dance life. "I've been a university professor for a long time, so I had this self-image as being sort of reserved. I thought a lot about how people perceive me as a professor—if they respect me, if they take me seriously. Then all of a sudden I started dancing, and people perceive that as a different kind of role—especially if you do blues dancing, because a lot of people look at it and go, 'Whoa, that's too sexy for me.' So there's a certain level of role incongruity that at first I didn't really want to acknowledge or deal with. But this is a fairly small city, so it's hard to not have people know what you do in your different roles in life. I've had to become more comfortable just saying, 'Yes, I'm a dancer.'"

Jill has had to explain what she gets out of the dance scene to her spouse, however. "It can sometimes be a challenge for my husband who may feel like a 'dance widower.' He is not a dancer, so my passion for blues dance means we sometimes take time away from each other, he for his hobbies and me for mine. It requires some balancing when your partner is not involved."

He recognizes however, the health benefits blues dancing has offered Jill. When asked how blues dancing makes her feel, she answered, "When I dance, I feel engaged, young, and powerful. I find it really calming and centering. It just has a kind of flow to it that I really embrace. It's really hard to put into words what it makes you feel. If I have trouble sleeping, I imagine blues dancing to a slow song—it makes me relax and slows my breathing."

In professorial fashion, Jill described blues music as "an encyclopedia of life lessons. It reminds me of how lucky I am, because the troubles in the music are not troubles in my own life. It also shows how people can find beauty in pain, and hope in loss."

The lesson Jill is most grateful to have learned through dance, however, is that she can find pleasure in social activities outside of work. "The thing about blues dancing is you can dance at any age and make friends you never imagined you would. Three or four years ago, if you had asked me if I was going to retire I probably would have said I don't think so, but now I'm ready to retire. When I get to the point where it's my retirement date, I'm going to retire. Although I still have stuff I want to write after that, I also want to dance. As long as I'm healthy, I will keep on dancing."

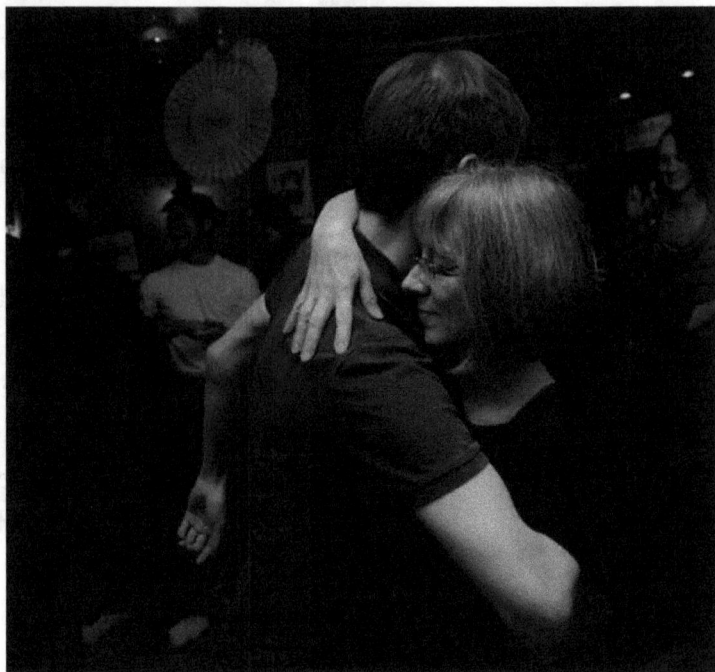

Photo by Patrick Fulgencio

A Community That Actually Cares

Tristan Brightman, Bristol, England

Tristan was the first person I interviewed for this book. After I made a call for stories at London's European Blues Invasion, he eagerly approached me with words that carried encouragement: "I have a story." He looked me in the eye with conviction. "You described your project, and I immediately felt you were speaking to me." It was affirmation that there were likely many others out there with stories of transformation through blues dancing—and that they would find their way to me.

He wasn't shy about opening up. His emotions had already been bled a couple of years before, when he found out his wife had been cheating on him.

"It was the worst time in my life," Tristan recalled. "It was really necessary for me to have something I could concentrate on that wasn't this world of feeling wronged and horrible." At first, he worked really hard to try to put their relationship back together, but it soon became clear it was beyond repair. He needed not only an activity to engage his mind but almost an entirely new social circle. Since his friends had equal ties to him and to his wife, they were reticent to get involved by discussing what had happened between them. "I had no one reaching out to support me. I lost the friends I had."

Tristan had begun Lindy Hop dancing on a casual basis. One night, there was a blues after-party, which he attended on a whim. He was attracted to the ability to connect directly with the music—and, soon, to the community. He became addicted to the blues. Soon after finding out about the infidelity, he was invited by an organizer to attend Livin' the Blues, a blues dance festival in Scotland. The event was on his wedding anniversary, and while he was trying to fix his marriage, he thought he would be unable to attend. He even joked with the organizer, "If I end up coming it will be because something terrible has happened." Less than two weeks later, he wrote her and asked if there was still space available at the event. He registered immediately and later that month packed his bags with a heavy but hopeful heart and headed to Glasgow.

"When I turned up there, I was almost an empty shell. Everything had been completely ripped away from me—which made it even easier to connect with people. I had no barriers. People would talk to me, and I'd just be me directly back."

Tristan shared that he was reasonably quick to pick up blues dancing, but it wasn't the dancing itself that permeated his memories of that first event—it was the people.

"Livin' the Blues felt like falling into this bed of love and friendliness and amazing people. The community did such a great job of looking after me, some of them without even knowing what was going on. Blues dancing gave me something to distract me from misery, and a new group of people to care about who cared about me. I genuinely believe that if it hadn't been for that, I'd be an alcoholic living with my parents, trying to piece together my life."

Tristan continued his involvement with the blues dance community upon his return to his home in Bristol, and the following year, he was asked to write the blessing for the Livin' the Blues festival. Tristan was honored to be a part of this small ceremony to bring the dancers together in celebration of the community. "I read my blessing, which was a thank-you poem about what the whole community meant to me. I managed to hold it together for the time I was in the circle, but after I read the poem, I went and broke down in the corner for a while. To be at that same event a year after my marriage ended and to be able to share what it had meant to me was so powerful."

Not long after his return, he was invited to attend another international blues festival—this one in the United States. Traveling that distance would have been out of the question in his earlier life, but the change of circumstance in his personal life—coupled with a pending change in his professional life—encouraged him to seriously consider the idea.

"With all the horror of the cheating and the breakup, I was not the best employee for a year. I'd go back to the office after a weekend at a blues event and be really confused as to why my boss didn't give me a hug. And at lunch time, we'd just go get a sandwich and then sit at our desks and do this work that wasn't really connected to anything in a direct and meaningful way. I would feel completely empty. At first, my employer was really understanding, but eventually they lost patience with me and offered me a severance package to leave the company."

Tristan now had nothing tying him down at home—even his lease was ending. "I realized it was probably the best time in my life to take time off for traveling." If he had needed another motivating factor to commit to the trip, he got it. Along with Anna Takkula, whose story is in the Body section, Tristan was a costume contest winner at the European Blues Invasion. His prize was a ticket to the Blues Recess event in northern Washington, where our paths would cross again, two months after the interview.

When we reconnected at Blues Recess, it was like I was meeting a slightly more evolved version of Tristan. In London, he was full of enthusiasm and excitement for what lay ahead—stored energy was emanating from his spirit, waiting to be released. In Washington, he had settled into the calm and comfort of "having arrived."

"When I was working, I had a limited amount of free time, so I couldn't really relax into anything I was doing. I'd go to the park, and it would be beautiful, but after fifteen minutes, I wouldn't be able to sit anymore—I'd have to get up and go do something. But here, I spend an hour sitting on my own at the top of the rock quarry, watching the sunlight on the water and just having a sense of peace. That's definitely one thing I want to take back into my life when I return—the ability to sit and just be in the moment."

Tristan still had another couple of months to travel before his journey would lead him back home, a time frame in which he hoped to figure out the next steps for his career. "My goal is to think about the broad pillars that I'm going to base my life on in the future. I know that I don't want to work five days in an office. It might happen, but while I'm here, I'll be thinking about ideas that might form the base for my future."

As the saying goes, one day he'll have to "go back to reality." But as he and I had discussed in London, the truth of what "reality" is is somewhat blurred. An outsider might say that an event like Livin' the Blues or Blues Recess—intentional communities based upon love and acceptance and human connection—is "removed from reality." But as Tristan shared from his experience, "nothing has ever felt more real."

"Reality" is that the connections and sensations experienced at dance events are carried on long after the event ends. Tristan convincingly declared at the end of our follow-up meeting, "This is a community I'm going to be in for as long as I've got legs." As if on cue, just down the path, we were able to discern Eros Salvatore—the dancer with a broken leg, whose story also appears in this book's Body section—hobbling along on his crutches. We gave each other a knowing look. "Well, maybe even without legs."

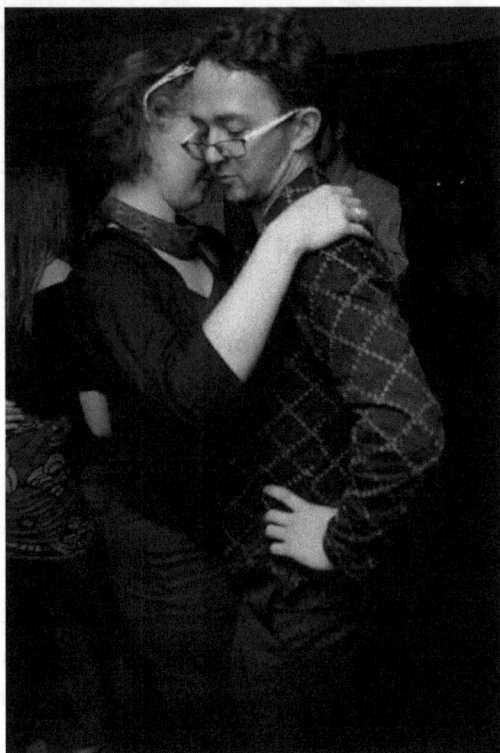

Photo by Kai Liesirova

Connecting Cultures

Vincent Wong, Vancouver, British Columbia, Canada

Finding a time to interview Vincent presented somewhat of a challenge—his professional and social lives were so busy. That was how I came to have an impromptu virtual tour of Vancouver's Classical Chinese Garden. Vincent serves as the community engagement manager of the organization and was making his rounds as we chatted via video conference. He also works in community engagement for Vancouver's Asian Film Festival, and maintains an active social dancing calendar. He prefers this kind of busy, however, to the busyness he had before dance.

"If I had not discovered the dance community, my life would be very different. I got started social dancing around 2008 when I was finishing a master's degree. My days involved a lot of sitting—hunkering down writing papers and working on my thesis. It was a bit like social seclusion, so as soon as my academic load lightened, I decided I would get involved in the community and reconnect with friends. I started participating in a lot of nonprofit organizations, and then a friend of mine was competing in a Lindy Hop competition, so I went out there to cheer her on."

Having been a member of a jazz orchestra in the past, he already felt connected to the big band music being played and so was inspired to take some Lindy

Hop classes. Within a year, what began as a light interest had evolved into regularly traveling to dance events. It was Seattle's Emerald City Blues Festival that sealed his devotion to blues—and his desire to use his community engagement skills to develop the local Vancouver blues and fusion scenes.

Vincent joined forces with some friends to organize a regular blues dance event of their own. "We held a dance at a bubble tea shop. It was a really cool, funky little space. We called the event Bubbles 'n' Blues—now it's called the Blues Café— and it has been running ever since."

The experience has been highly rewarding. "The people who come are always really warm, welcoming, enthusiastic people. They say thank you for putting it on—there's all this love and appreciation and so many friendships get made by coming out to the event." The dance is no longer exclusively blues—it has emerged into more of a fusion event, attracting members from the salsa, tango, zook, and kizomba communities— which runs parallel to various social and cultural crossovers that Vincent has come to appreciate and promote.

At the root of his character is the desire to break down barriers—not just on the dance floor. "When I tell someone that I'm involved in organizing a dance event, the first question I get is the one everybody in the blues dance community gets: 'You can dance to blues?!' But then I get the exclamations: 'That's really interesting—tell me more.' It's a great conversation starter and a way to share with people the world of blues or Lindy or partner dancing. When you tell non-dancers about the community, often they're impressed to find out that there's something you can go out to do in the evening that's not bopping to loud bass or getting drunk."

Vincent is passionate not just about sharing the social community of dance with others but about inspiring people to learn more about history. "Blues and Lindy Hop have histories going back decades and just learning the art form gives you a connection to that history. It's a gateway to learn about the past. I work in a classical Chinese garden because I really enjoy learning the roots of where we come from—whether it's our own personal roots or the roots of where we live.

"Vancouver is very multicultural, very cosmopolitan, so it has given me a connection to both Western cultures and my roots in Hong Kong and China. I find that social dance gives me a little bit of the same because you're dancing with the art form of today's world with today's people, but at the same time you're learning to appreciate some of that connection between history and today—what still survives and persists and is still relevant."

One of the ways Vincent has been able to connect to his roots in China is via Vancouver's active martial arts community. He has practiced Wushu—an exhibition and full-contact sport—and participated in lion dance performances around the city. "Lion dance is very different than social dance, although it *is* done in partners—you have two people per lion costume." Vincent smiled at his attempt to find correlation between the two dance styles, before landing on a deeper connection.

"One of the reasons I found partner dancing to be such a logical step for me is because of the foundations that I learned in martial arts. I learned how to have strong stances—how to be stable, how to have good balance, and how to hold my body. Wushu is a very performance-oriented martial art with fluid movements, which very easily correlated to blues and fusion movements. It doesn't necessarily give you the same appreciation of musical rhythm, but I had that from having been a musician."

Vincent has used his experience as a musician to cross social barriers as well. "I've been playing violin since I was four years old. Occasionally I still play electric violin with a local Art Rock band, but not often. However, I had the unexpected special honor to perform at the Urban Blues Recess event in Portland in 2011. There was a workshop where everyone was invited to bring his or her instruments. I brought my violin, as did one of the other dancers. We hit it off and jammed well together, so one night after the workshop, we were playing near the tent area. A musician for the event heard us jamming and invited us to be in the show that night." I could see the excitement of that night relived on Vincent's face as he told me the story.

His love for live music runs deep—just as deep as his love for dance. I got the impression that in

Vincent's version of a perfect world, everyone would share his interest in music, in dance, and in breaking any barrier that keeps people apart. At the very least, it would keep him from experiencing the highly uncomfortable position most partner dancers know well: "When I go to a really great live music show and there is nobody in the room who knows how to partner dance—oh my god, that is so hard!" Vincent rolled his head back, and his eyes furrowed in distress.

He is certainly doing his part to ensure those experiences occur less frequently. "I always try to find some opportunity to share dance with others. I would love for other people to be able to learn this wonderful art form that allows people to make connections with other people, with the past, and with music and the arts in different ways. After all, the very heart of culture and heritage lies in bringing people together and creating strong communities, and that—plus the sheer fun of the art form—is what makes dancing truly worthwhile."

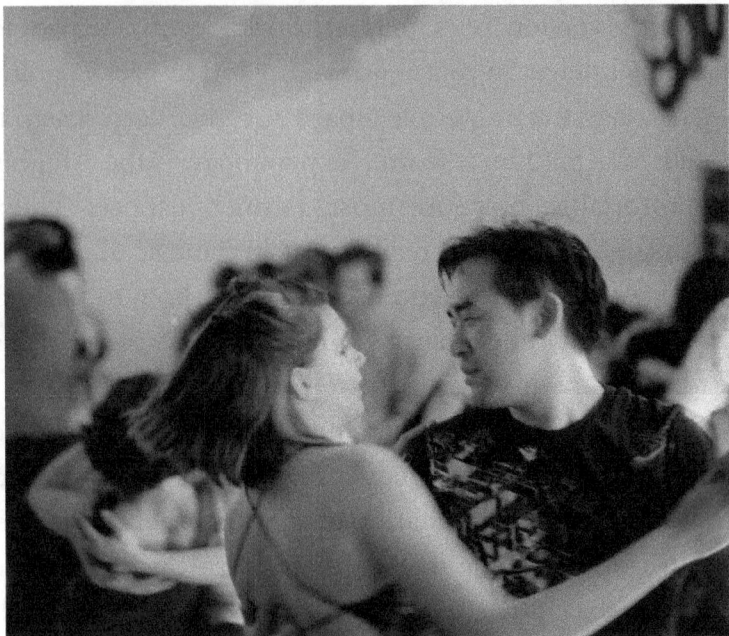

Photo by Drew Tronvig

From Me to King of the World

Alberto Escalante, Vitoria, Spain

A lberto reached out to me because his friends told him to. In his words, "I am not sure if my story is interesting, but the blues community has taught me to believe in your friends, and all of them think I should talk with you." He sent me his website, and I read his bio: "May 23, 2009 at 4:30 pm (a date and time I could never forget), I discovered what has become my passion: blues dancing." That settled it. I didn't know what his story entailed, but I knew that if he had such a memory, we had to talk.

We met over video conference, and it did not take long for me to discover that Alberto is a man robust not just in body but in charm. In fact, it is that quality that led Alberto from a more solitary life of "work, sleep" to a rich social life of "work, sleep, dance." He exuded warmth with every breath—and with every boisterous laugh he released after each question I presented. At times, we stumbled through communication. Basque being his first language, Spanish his second, we spoke in his third, English. But the essence of his love for the blues, and his desire to share it with others, was never mistaken.

"My story isn't so special," he again reminded me. "I just love to dance. But I can tell you what I feel with blues dancing. I feel something special. When you are dancing with someone and you feel them very close to you, I can't explain what that is for me. I feel something warm. I tell people blues dancing is easy— you just have to feel the music. Just come as you are and feel the music."

Alberto was not new to dancing at the time he became aware of the contemporary blues dance scene. He had already been dancing tango for fifteen years, and Lindy Hop for three years. When he first heard that a dance called blues existed, his first reaction was a common one. "Blues? Blues is the music. I knew the music but I didn't know the dance at all. Then when I saw people dancing after a Lindy Hop workshop, I noticed something special—that was how I dance! Even when I'm dancing Lindy Hop or tango to a slow song. I didn't know it was called blues."

Despite implementing the blues dance aesthetic when dancing other styles, Alberto found little opportunity to dance to blues music with partners who knew about the style. "I live in a small city where it's difficult to dance. There are only five blues dancers here, so if we want to study the dance, we use YouTube."

Or they travel. "If I want to dance blues, I have to take a flight or probably two flights. The airport here is not too big, so you have to fly to Madrid, Barcelona, Paris, London, or Frankfurt. Actually, I know all the time schedules for all the flights from Bilbao, and when I arrive there, I always see people I know because I travel so much for dancing."

Alberto's blues skills were able to advance enough that he could begin teaching the dance himself. Now he is one of the dancers seen on YouTube that others have begun to recognize and study. He has become accustomed to strangers approaching him and saying, "You're the guy who dances! Can you teach me to dance?"

His Lindy Hop classes are more heavily advertised since the dance has more popularity in Spain; however, his joy at being approached to teach dance reaches considerable more depth when someone asks him about blues. "When someone who has seen me blues dancing asks me, 'Would you mind teaching me blues?' I say *yesssssss*." Alberto's face lit up, as though his new student had uncovered his secret.

Word must be getting around. "I have to put a new post on my website that says I'm completely full for the next six months. I'm very proud of that." Although Alberto loves sharing what he knows and is passionate about helping others, he has no aspiration to be a competitive or professional dancer. The defining moment for that decision was at a competition in Berlin.

"I finished the competition, and I did not pass to the final. There were four judges, and three came to me and told me, 'We voted for you to be in the finals,' but the other judge said, 'No, anybody except him.' In the beginning I felt sad, but then I realized, actually, I don't mind not being in the final. I feel so nice with myself and my dance. At that moment, I decided I don't have to be a professional. I want to just enjoy it."

What's important to Alberto is not only how the dance feels for himself but how it feels for his dance partner. "I realized at some point that I have to dance for my follow—not with her, but for her. A lot of people have told me they enjoy dancing with me, and that is so special to me. That's what matters."

That's not the only reward Alberto has received from blues dancing. "When I discovered blues, my life started to change. In that moment, I noticed there was something different in me—I became more social. I could express myself to the people who were dancing with me, express who I am. For example, I love being playful when I dance blues. I love to make people laugh. It makes me feel like there was a part of me that probably had been there for years, but I had not shown."

Dancing—and not being afraid to be himself—led to him meeting his girlfriend. "I have a girlfriend who loves to dance blues. Somebody asked me if I could have a girlfriend who did not dance, and the answer was hard, because the truth is…probably not. I live for that. And I don't want to change my life. Dancing is so important in my life. Now I have a girlfriend, and I'm really happy with her. I've started teaching with her in some places, and it is really, really good."

That's a feat he once thought unlikely. When I asked him to tell me about one of his most powerful moments dancing, he let out a loud exclamation. "Whoa! There are so many. The first special one was when I had to stop living with my now ex-girlfriend, which was really hard for me because we were together ten years. I started thinking, 'Okay, I'm thirty-seven years old; I'm quite fat—it's true; I think it's not going to be easy to meet girls.' I went to a dance festival in France after the breakup, and there I met a girl. And actually, it was really, really easy to kiss again. I remember that moment well."

It's no wonder it's easy for Alberto to connect with women on the dance floor, considering this philosophy: "I never say no to a girl if she asks me to dance...Maybe if I'm really tired. When I start feeling like I'm not doing my best when I'm dancing, it's time to go. If I can't do my best for that girl, why should that girl not get the best of me like the other girl? I'm not comfortable with that, so it's time to go; tomorrow will be a better day to dance with me."

Alberto sometimes fears he isn't as good at offering his family the same time and attention he gives his dance partner. "After a year and a half of traveling every weekend, I started to feel bad, because I have my family here who wants to see me. So I decided at least to leave one weekend each month where I don't travel to go dancing."

Even so, his family still worries when he travels so much. Alberto has a strategy to remedy that, however. "My mother got worried about me when I started traveling so much for dancing. Actually, I don't have my family on Facebook because I don't want them to be like, 'Where are you now?' One time my mother called and asked, 'Hey, how are you? How is the weather?' It was in December of last year, and it was snowing, crazy snowing—because I was in Moscow! And I knew that in Basque country it was nice weather, so I told her, 'Ahhhh it's very humid.' I didn't want her to worry about me."

Even though his mother may not like her son being gone so much, Alberto can tell his mother is proud of his dancing. "My parents came to a swing event two years ago at the main theater here in Vitoria. I made a small show dancing blues, and when I finished, my father didn't say a lot—he was like, 'He's happy; that's good.' My mother first said, 'It was nice,' but then she noticed there were a lot of people that came up to me and said, 'Wow, Alberto! You were amazing!' So my mother thought, 'Okay, people are saying that—that's quite good.'"

His mother's recognition of his talent backfired in one particular—but playful—way. "That year, I went to two or three family weddings. Here they have the main meal and then a dance—nothing fancy, just paso doble or something easy. And it's funny, my mother says to the family, 'You can dance with Alberto because he dances a lot.' And I said, 'Mom, I don't dance to this kind of music. I don't dance at all like this!'" But his reply went unheeded. "A woman who was about seventy-five years old came to me and said, 'Alberto, let's dance! Cha-cha-cha! Salsa!'" Alberto threw his head back in annoyance but maintained a joyful composure at the memory.

Despite the social hardship his family sometimes brings to his life, Alberto would not trade his home for anything. "I want to live here near my family and friends. I am a computer engineer, so if I wanted only to work, San Jose in California is perfect. But I don't just want to work. I have a huge community here now through dance."

Alberto doesn't even have to travel to see that community. He brings the party to his home—a flat constructed exclusively for him. "For me, my flat is my life. I wanted to design it around what it is important to me. You're going to laugh, but it's the truth: I love having baths. So I decided I needed a bath for me, which is not easy—I'm a big guy. So I went to the south of Spain; I traveled nine hours to discover a place that could make a huge bathtub designed for me."

And that's not all. "The other thing that I love is cooking. Most people from the Basque country love cooking, so my kitchen is large. I also love cinema, so I have this big screen. And the main thing is I love dancing, so I decided to make a house designed especially for that. Here I have a special floor that you can dance on comfortably." At this point, I asked Alberto if I could have a virtual tour of his flat. The design—and his enthusiasm for it—had me intrigued.

The tour concluded with Alberto's finishing touch—a strobe light and stereo system used exclusively for dance parties. I could imagine how fun a dance party at Alberto's would be—not just because of the home's design but more because of Alberto himself.

His girlfriend agrees. "My girlfriend tells me that I'm a donut, because when I go to a party, everyone comes." Being the life of the party is a role Alberto now cherishes. "It's theater, in a way. I feel like an actor in some moments, playing King of the World." Lest anyone misinterpret this bequeathed role for ego, Alberto finished, "But I'm still me."

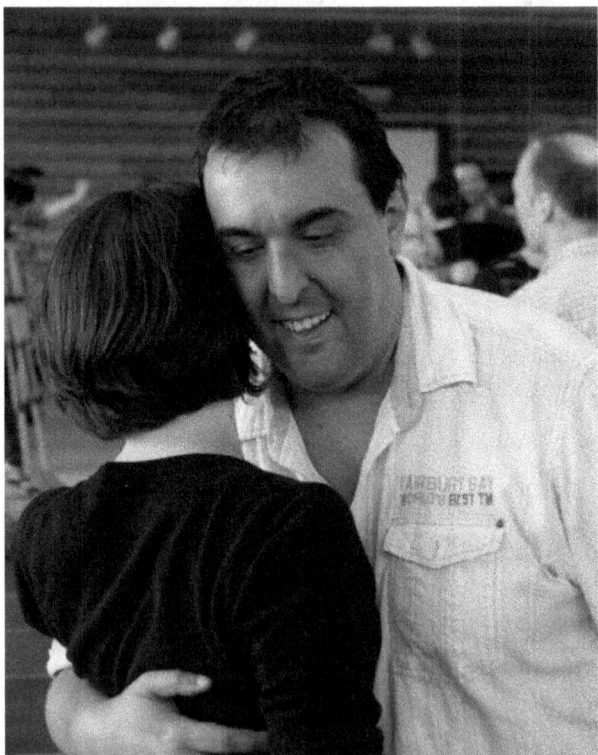

Photo by Kai Liesirova

VI
SINGING THE BLUES

Music is by no means a requirement in order to dance, but it is often the inspiration. Just as some people are called to move as soon as a blues rhythm hits, others are called to sing or pick up a musical instrument. Still others are inspired to do both.

Some contributors to this section are both blues dancers and blues musicians; they feel equally comfortable stepping down from the stage for a dance and stepping right back up to perform. Or in some cases, dancing and singing on stage at the same time. Others are musicians who believe they have two left feet or simply aren't comfortable with the intimacy of dancing. Delving into dance leads to heightened vulnerability for some, whereas playing dance music is where they shine.

Whether or not the two areas complement each other in one individual, it cannot be denied that they enrich each other in general. What I found interesting is that several of the musicians in this section had been playing blues music for years without knowing that a parallel dance scene existed. Once they experienced playing for a blues dance crowd, their minds were somewhat blown—they had never played for an audience so attentive and engaged. Nor had they played to a crowd so appreciative of slow blues songs—which the dance form tends to require. More than one artist described the experience as "heavenly."

I remain curious, therefore, why more blues musicians don't seek out this hungry market. I suppose it's mostly due to lack of awareness that it exists. I hope this book helps bring awareness to the dance community. As for the dancers, I hope they are inspired to seek out more opportunities to dance to live music. Not only can it be argued that a greater depth of experience and joy occurs when the energy between dancer and musician play off each other, but supporting the careers of blues musicians is what is going to make this music stick around. And by extension, also the dance.

The Blues Is My Home

Kevin Selfe, Portland, Oregon, USA

Although I had enjoyed seeing Kevin perform at both dance and non-dance events many times over the years, I had never introduced myself. Perhaps it's a result of having worked in the music industry, but I tend to make an assumption that people in show business don't have time for fans. In some cases, that is most certainly true—but in Kevin's case, I witnessed the opposite. He is always making the rounds before and after his gigs, offering gratitude and camaraderie to those who support his music.

Perhaps that is why, with my book as its own introduction, I ultimately felt comfortable asking Kevin to sit down for an interview. I shared with him the scope of the project and invited him to discuss it further over coffee. His was the first interview I held for this particular section, and I was somewhat nervous. I need not have been; I'd prepared a handwritten list of questions to use as prompts, and although his nature is on the quiet side, if he's talking about his passion, he does so with ease.

He began by telling me how he came to play guitar. "In middle school, we had to take band class and pick an instrument to play. I picked trumpet. I picked up guitar in high school because I wanted to do something else musical; I had a friend who had a guitar and I thought it was cool. So my dad bought me a cheap used one to see if I would stick with it. I took a couple of lessons and taught myself the rest."

His exposure to blues music came through his own musical exploration. "I remember hearing this song by AC/DC called 'Baby, Please Don't Go.' I thought it was really cool—it sounded so different than what they usually did. I started looking through the liner notes, and I learned that they didn't write the song—J. Williams did. Who is J. Williams? He's not in the band. So I started researching it, and I found out it was written by a guy named Big Joe Williams, a Delta blues musician who played this nine-string bastardized guitar. I got a copy of the original, and it didn't sound anything like what I was used to hearing. It was just acoustic, really raw. It was fascinating to me; that stuck with me."

Kevin didn't stray from his love of heavy rock just yet, however. Another light had to go off—which happened a couple of years later, when his college roommate put on a record from his music collection. "It was this really dark, eerie voice and guitar that just grabbed a hold of me. I came to find out it was 'Smokestack Lighting' by Howlin' Wolf. I was nineteen at the time, and I still remember how I felt when I heard that song. I can just see the whole room and everything; it was a really powerful experience. After that, I started getting into all kinds of blues—Muddy Waters, Elmore James, John Lee Hooker."

Kevin's roommate was a bass player, making it convenient to hold impromptu jam sessions in their room. If he wasn't in class, he was likely playing guitar.

"I was shy, really shy until I was about twenty-one or twenty-two. So when I went from a really small high school to a huge university, I got swallowed up. I just went to school and studied and played guitar—that was it. When I went home for summer break, I was in the basement eight to ten hours a day, just playing."

After graduating college with a meteorology degree, he returned to his hometown in Virginia and began playing in blues jams and open mics. It didn't take long for him to decide not to pursue his major; he wanted to play the blues. He picked up various side jobs to support himself, always keeping that ultimate goal in mind.

"I worked in a steel plant for a couple years—which was really hard—and at the same time I was a high school football coach, which is how I got into my very first band. I was coaching some of the kids on the team who had a little garage band. They asked me to help them out in a gig and one thing led to another until I was asked to audition for the Fat Daddy Band there in Roanoke."

At the time, Kevin was working the evening shift at a coffee shop, which conflicted with the band's schedule. He transitioned to working at a music store during the day to accommodate the band's growing popularity, but retail wasn't his forte. Finally, he ran all the numbers and realized he could survive just making music. "My last day at work was January 5, 2001. That was my last day job. It was scary, but I knew I at least wanted to give it a try. I've been doing solely music for a living for fifteen years now. It's still scary."

He did come to realize, however, that if he wanted to continue to grow as a blues musician, he would likely have to leave Roanoke. "I'd been playing in bands in Virginia for almost ten years, and I felt like I was outgrowing the scene there. There were only a handful of really good musicians there, so if I needed someone to fill in at a gig, the second- or third-call guys weren't very strong.

"So I began researching communities that had good blues scenes; the first thing I did was look to see where the biggest blues societies were for musicians and blues music, and Portland had one of the biggest. So I flew out here to check it out; I got off the plane, and a couple hours later, I was already playing in a jam."

Kevin didn't know anyone in Portland, but he began to make connections by attending local blues jams. It wasn't long before he started to pick up paid gigs, an opportunity he still feels grateful for. "There are very few cities in the country where you'd be able to do what I do."

Part of the reason Kevin is able to do what he does is due to the support of the blues dance community. Interestingly, he wasn't even aware that this community existed before he moved to Portland. "There was no blues dancing scene on the East Coast, just people who showed up to our gigs and…'danced'— it wasn't pretty, let's just put it that way. It was a lot of drunk people moving around."

His introduction to the blues dance scene in Portland began when opening up for another local blues band. "They got the dancers out to do a demonstration between sets, and I watched a little of the lesson. I was intrigued by the fact that there were all these younger people who liked blues; it wasn't the usual demographic of forty-to-sixty-year-olds. I was impressed; my only experience with something like that was seeing people swing dance, so at first I was trying to put blues dancing into this swing dancing box, but then I noticed it was different. We'd play a faster song, and they wouldn't dance. I thought, 'Why aren't they dancing? I thought these were swing dancers.' It didn't make any sense."

He liked what he saw, however. "I would watch and just be mesmerized by these people doing this slow, sensual, almost sexual dance right in front of all these people. I was pretty fascinated by it. It seemed like this really sensual experience that two people were sharing together, but then they would have another partner. I was like, 'How does that work?!' Usually when you share those kinds of moments with someone, it's someone you are intimate with, and I had a hard time in the very beginning wrapping my brain around how people could share these three-to-five-minute sensual experiences and then move on."

Kevin would find out how it worked by befriending some of the blues dancers. Through these relationships, he was hired to perform at one of the weekly dance events.

"I was so excited and nervous and scared. Before the gig, I ended up going to one of the dances just to watch. The thing that struck me was that they were dancing to deejayed music. I thought, 'Why are they dancing to deejayed music, when there are all these great bands out here?' I couldn't get over that, until I started to realize that most of them didn't know there was a live blues music scene or how to access it. I'd say, 'I play at Duff's Garage,' and they'd say, 'Where's that?'" Kevin gave a look of incredulousness that the venue he spoke of was only five blocks from the weekly dance event, but many blues dancers had never even heard of it.

The reason for that is due in part to the style of blues music played at such venues. Kevin came to learn that dancers only respond to particular tempos and beats.

"In the beginning, I would just play my regular show, but then I realized that some of the things I was playing were not suitable for blues dancing. I began to go watch other bands play for dancers and listen to what was being deejayed between sets. There was some trial and error, but then I got to a format."

He began to leave up-tempo songs off his sets, focusing on slower-to-medium-tempo songs with a pulse. "It has to have a pulse, and that doesn't mean it has to be with an instrument either. I used to think that if a song doesn't have a strong beat, then people wouldn't dance to it, but that's not the case. It has to do with the vocals; the vocals can have a really strong rhythm to them that draws you in. I learned that by playing solo shows—just me and the guitar. It's been really good for me to learn what was resonating with the dancers; it's so inspiring to see them connect to the music."

What Kevin has learned by playing for blues dancers crosses over into his regular bar sets, as well as what makes it onto his new albums. "In the bar scene, not a lot of people get up and dance. So I started playing the songs blues dancers would get up and dance to, and other people would get up and dance too. I've noticed that I'm a lot more mindful of the tempos when I'm writing now; I still write some faster songs, but overall I use more dancer-friendly tempos."

Kevin's curiosity about the dance extended beyond what to play for his audience; despite his shyness, he eventually gave in to trying blues dancing out himself. The impetus was the end of his relationship with a blues dancer he'd been dating. "When we broke up, I missed all the friends that I made in the dance scene. I felt like not only did I lose the relationship, I lost a lot of the people I was in contact with, so I wanted to learn how to blues dance to stay involved with the community, not just from the stage.

"I took lessons for six months. I can remember practicing in front of the mirror; my apartment had this studio space, and I would practice for hours." Just when he started getting the hang of it, however, a painful experience led Kevin to redirect his energy back to playing music.

"I was playing the Waterfront Blues Festival six months after the breakup. I was up on stage singing 'Dancing Girl,' which was a song I'd written about my ex-girlfriend. I look up, and there she was, dancing right in front of me with another man. I wanted to leave, but I couldn't go anywhere or do anything—there were five thousand people there. That was the day that I said, 'I'm not going to dance anymore.' It was too painful. So I decided that if I was going to spend a lot of time practicing something that it was going to be my music."

As so often happens with the creative arts, however, something beautiful came out of that experience. "I ended up writing a song about it and putting it on my next album. It's called 'Blues Is My Home.' It's about healing. It's the only song where it's just me and the guitar. The only way I knew to express myself and get that pain out was by writing, by putting it down. There's something about it that makes me feel better; it feels like I'm putting this pain toward something that's good. I almost didn't put it on the record—I was too scared—but I think that song gets played more than any other song of mine."

Aside from writing it down, I asked Kevin what he felt was particular about blues music that generated the experience of healing. He replied, "There's something in the music itself; you have to separate the lyrical writing, which is cathartic, from something that's deeper and more primal about the actual sounds of blues music.

"For me, it starts with just me and the guitar. When I'm feeling *really* bad, I pull out this little old National steel guitar I have and my slide. There's something about those in between notes on a scale that you can't really get on a piano or a regular fretting instrument—you have to have a slide somehow. It's almost ambiguous, you can't really decipher what it is at times." Kevin paused for a great length of time in order to gain more clarity before continuing.

"There's this theory about how sound through an instrument resonates through your body cavity. The human body is really sensitive to vibration; it even goes back to when you're in the womb and you hear the vibration of your mother or father's voice. It's a really primal instinct that we have, and it's really healing. There are times when I'm just so tired and down, that I'll be leaning over my guitar—almost hugging it—playing a note, hearing it vibrate, and it really calms me."

Another experience that elevates Kevin's mood is playing for an audience tuned in to his performance. Often, he said, he plays for people who are distracted in one way or another—by their phones, by ordering at the bar, by conversation with their friends. "But when I play for dancers, I feel more connected to the audience. I like to interact with them. I'll hit these accents and do stops, or bring the intensity up and down really quickly, just playing with the dancers. I'll notice what they are responding to and just go from there."

As I mentioned in the introduction, there can be an intense energetic exchange between musicians and dancers. One experience I feel grateful to have witnessed—the one that inspired this book—is one Kevin played a part in. He had performed at Portland's Rose City Blues Festival Friday night and was attending the event the following night to see his friend, Curtis Salgado—whose story closes this book—, perform. He ended up coming to the band's rescue. "I kind of had a feeling he had no idea what this dance event was all about. Curtis is an incredible performer, but I knew if he went into it like I did when I started, it wasn't going to go over as well as he would have wanted. So I went there to give him some pointers—I told him what tempos to stay away from, told him not to make their songs so long, and so on."

Curtis realized his band was in over their heads. He made the quick decision to ask Kevin to sit in with his band during his set. "He asked me to call out the songs—tell them what the tempo was and everything, so I was helping him through that process. And what ended up happening that night I'd never seen before. There were a few hundred people there, mostly partner dancing, but then people starting breaking off. There must have been twenty to thirty people up front solo dancing. I'd never seen them do that. I was like, 'Wow! These people are into the music, just connecting with their bodies.' I wanted to figure out how to have that experience with my band."

Kevin played close attention to what inspired that reaction at Curtis's show, and realized it had to do with the vocals. He started taking vocal lessons from

Curtis's vocal coach. "Curtis had been hammering that home to me. He was like, 'You can be a great player, and you can write great songs, but if you can't sing, your audience is not going to connect with you.' So that's what I've really been trying to work on—figuring out how to connect more with the dancers. I get excited every time we play for dancers. It's my favorite thing to do."

In reality, he's not sure if there's a sustainable community—and therefore career—for blues music. "The future of blues music…it's scary. It really is. I see a lot of great musicians out there but no demand for the music. There are not a lot of people going out to listen to it. More important, there aren't any younger people going out to listen to it. The age group that goes out to hear blues…I hate to say it, but they're dying off. The little bit of hope that I have is that the blues dance community is all younger people who are interested and like blues music."

He had another idea of what could reignite interest in the music. "There has to be some sort of shift in mainstream music for it to really work. It doesn't have to be a big shift. In the '80s, it was Stevie Ray Vaughn; in the '60s it was the Rolling Stones and the Beatles who brought out this revolution of blues music, so every twenty years it looks like something happens. I see it so close—with the Black Keys and the White Stripes—so close to what a lot of us do musically that there could be just a little shift for the media to change the way it sees blues. That's something I've thought about a lot. I think about it almost every day."

I made the assumption Kevin also regularly thought about what he'd do if he could no longer make a living as a musician. He confirmed, "I ask myself that question all the time, just because of the state of blues music right now, and I have no idea. I'm hoping that if the time came when I did need to do something else, I would know."

In the meantime, Kevin is going to keep on singing and playing—in the only way he can. "All my songs have a story behind them. I think that's what makes good songs, it's what the blues is about. I think if you can't tell your own story, you're not a blues musician. I play some covers just like everybody else does, but when I can tell my personal story in musical form, that's what I feel gives me validation as a blues musician. Nobody else can sing my songs like I do. That's what makes me me, what makes me authentic. That's what we have to be in all this: we have to be authentic."

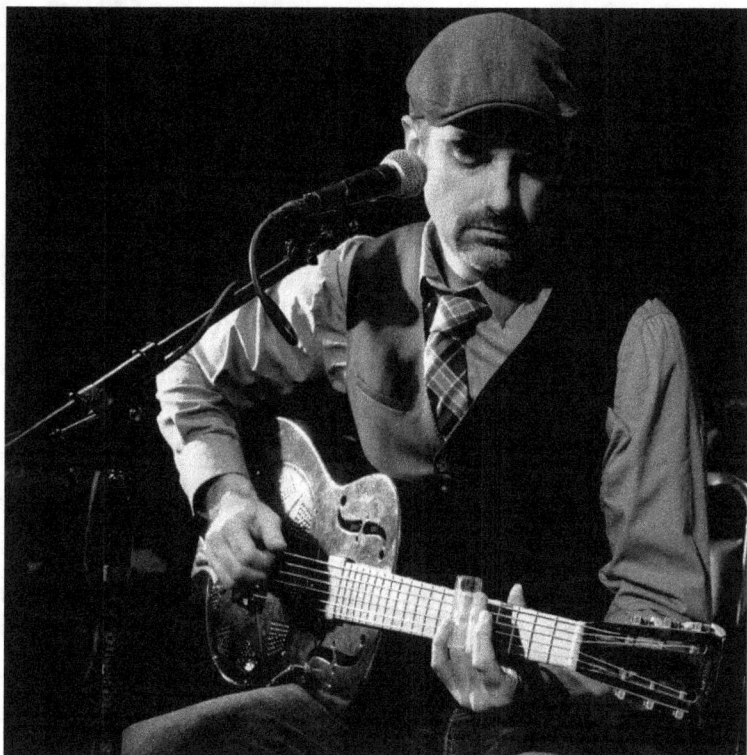

Photo by Eric Frommer

The Song Tells Me Everything I Need to Know

Velody, Manchester, England

I made various announcements through UK blues dance channels, inviting members of the scene to be interviewed for this book. Velody reached out to me after I'd already returned to Nashville, where I was residing for a few months. We discussed holding an interview through videocam, but it turned out we'd get to meet in person after all—Velody would soon be traveling to Nashville to teach a blues workshop. So it is in the dance world; sooner or later, paths do cross—in one country or another.

Especially if you travel as much as Velody. By performing in her blues band, teaching blues dance, or attending a dance event for pleasure, she's liable to be in someplace different every time you hear from her. A few months after our interview, I saw her in my home city of Portland.

"I'm very grateful that blues has afforded me the opportunity to tour the world as much as I do, particularly around the States. It's funny—before I came over, one of my students in Manchester said to me: 'You're going to teach blues over there? Isn't that kind of like taking cheese to the French?' I smiled and saw what he was saying; however, having had the privilege to grow up with this music, to sing blues for years and train in this style of dance for seven years, I feel like there's a contribution I can make. And I'm so grateful that other people think so too."

At a favorite coffee shop of mine in downtown Nashville, we met up after her workshop and before an evening out dancing at a local blues bar. I learned Velody grew up listening to singers such as Billie Holiday, Nina Simone, and Ella Fitzgerald. She said, "I found that vocal gymnastics like scatting didn't really do much for me, whereas the more earthy style of singers like Bessie Smith or Billie Holiday resonated deeply. In terms of my singing, both my parents told me of my murmuring and gurgling away tunefully when I was very small, way before I began talking. I started writing songs when I was ten—I still have most of my lyrics sheets saved at home! I'd experiment with blues phrasing and the call-and-response that blues is known for."

Although Velody stated that there was never a time when she didn't move to music, it wasn't until her adult life—while performing at burlesque nights—that she discovered there was much more to partner dancing than Fred Astaire and Ginger Rogers. She witnessed Lindy Hop dance first and had been enrolled in classes for three weeks before she heard about an upcoming blues workshop in Cambridge, England, featuring Dave Madison—featured in this book's opening section. "That was April 2008. It's still really clear in my mind to this day. I was excited to find a vocabulary of movement to something that had been a part of my life for so long."

Velody got even more excited when she walked into the social dance that night. "I had only done a little bit of dancing in a studio at that point, with six to twelve people in class. Then I walked into a beautiful church hall full of dancers swinging out to a live band. It absolutely blew me away. After that, I never looked back."

She is able to articulate now what it is about the music and the dance that drew her in. "Blues has a simplicity but also infinite layers within it. It has a storytelling aspect and an edge, or rawness to it. Everything is stripped back, and it's just you—whether you are a guy with a guitar, one voice singing, or you are just moving to a song. For me, when I'm dancing blues, the song tells me everything I need to know."

At the time, Manchester did not have its own blues dance scene. Velody expanded her dance repertoire by attending Lindy exchanges around the United Kingdom that had late-night blues rooms. As is often the case at dance events, however, as a follow, she would find herself on the sidelines due to the imbalance between leads and follows. One night at a Lindy exchange in the autumn of 2008, she decided she wasn't going to sit out all night at dances anymore. "Quite probably it was rather shoddy and without much finesse, but I decided I was going to lead on the social dance floor. I think the advantage I had, though, was being a musician and a singer; I already felt rhythms and phrasing in the music."

So perhaps Velody's first dance student was herself, but before long she branched out to teach others. "For about six to nine months, I demoed alongside my first Lindy and balboa teacher. I had studied martial arts—specifically tai chi—for seven years before that, so I was used to guiding students and describing physical movement. From tai chi I learned good balance: you have to be fully grounded and have conscious awareness of where your weight is. Tai chi is also a slow and purposeful discipline, so I brought that to my blues teaching."

Velody recognized that although she was still relatively new to dance, she was aware of her strengths. "As soon as I understand something, I'm able to articulate it in both technical and layperson terms. I knew I wasn't as accomplished as some of the more experienced dancers, but what I was able to do well was articulate the basics of how to move correctly, paving a clear path for our students. I still focus on simple terms in my workshops today as I don't like to obstruct learning with overtly technical language."

Her musical background helped her gain a teaching advantage as well. "In music, we have strict guidelines like what key or tempo to play in, but it's up to you how to style it. It's the same in dance; if you're leading, you have to be clear with what you're inviting your partner to do, but then as the follow it's up to you how you style it. Within the confines of what you've been invited to do, there are a lot of possibilities in how you dance it."

Velody's martial art and musical perspective, combined with her growing skills in teaching and leading, led her to be able to gather a few local dancers in her community and host an introduction to blues workshop. Interest grew from there, and since 2011 Velody has been able to grow a successful career dedicated to singing, dancing, and teaching blues, Lindy, and balboa—often doing them all at the same event!

"One of my passions is to play for dancers. It's kind of a niche market; our songs need to be of a certain length and have clear phrasing. They need to have a clear ending too, so dancers can say thank you to each other and move to the next dance. As a dancer, I pick up ways I can improve my band's sets for dancers; it gives you the edge if you understand both disciplines. I thought about this a lot when making my recent album *Faces*."

Velody has similarly high goals for her teaching, as well. "I want to help people free themselves a little bit, to bring it back to the fundamentals—the music, you, and your partner. Even more important is to remember what brings us here, the love of an awesome groove or getting to share movement with someone else.

"That's why I enjoy teaching regularly. I get to check in and do a quick audit on how I'm delivering for the group. Hopefully I'm equipping people to go forward—not as versions of me or my individual style but as better versions of themselves. That's the open learning environment that I create, rather than teaching moves, moves, moves, which people get elsewhere."

Aside from what she hopes to impart to her audience or her students, Velody has received her own share of life lessons from dancing. "One of the things I like about blues is, like tai chi, it slows me down a little bit. I'm generally quite a fast-paced person, and after living on the road for twenty months, I learned the importance of giving my body (and mind) recovery time afterward. Time to allow my body to heal. If you're a teacher, a musician, or a traveling dancer, energy management is hugely important. As a performer, there's a lot of adrenaline going around your body, so allowing time for recovery ensures that your body's energy levels—and therefore your career and your contribution—are sustainable. That was an important lesson for me."

Dance has played a part in Velody's healing process in other ways as well. One of the most powerful examples of this took place at a dance event in London. "I had been in a long-time relationship that had just ended, and I think I was still trying to come to terms with what had happened. I was at one of the late-night dances, and it was somewhere between three and five in the morning. I was following in close embrace, and maybe it was the song or how safe I felt in the embrace, but I suddenly found myself in a flood of tears. I was like, 'Wow, this is interesting. Keep dancing; hopefully my partner won't be freaked out.'" Velody laughed gently at the memory before pausing and continuing. "It was a really powerful healing moment for me; I realized the grief for this loss had not been consciously acknowledged...but was waiting to be acknowledged."

Music has always been an outlet for Velody's emotion, and dancing is just another way to inspire that release. "When I'm dancing blues, there's a definite moment when I let the music wash over me. I actually feel it come through my heart and go back outward. Everything I need in order to dance is in the song."

It isn't only the music Velody referred to—it's the lyrics. "I'm a lyricist, so it's very rare that a dodgy lyric will get past me. It's great to see who is really listening to the words at gigs. I'll sometimes throw in a curve ball to check if dancers are listening to what we're doing or if they are just doing their basic steps. It's fine if they are just doing their steps, but I like people testing me too. We do one completely improvised number at every gig—inviting people to heckle us with content—and then it's my job to make sense of all the parts. The more challenging the heckle, the more it tests our mettle! I like the interaction."

Whether it's in her audience or her students, Velody loves observing transformation. "I've certainly witnessed my students loosening up and tuning in to the music more. What excites me is when I can see the lightbulb ignite—that breakthrough moment when a lead starts to realize the power in simplicity (rather than constantly aiming for complexity). Or when a follow really owns the space they're in and can wait without worrying over what's coming next. Blues music itself originates from a time when everything certainly wasn't rosy, but it's pioneers had ownership of the moment: 'we have right here, right now, let's truly live it.' That spirit needs to remain with us."

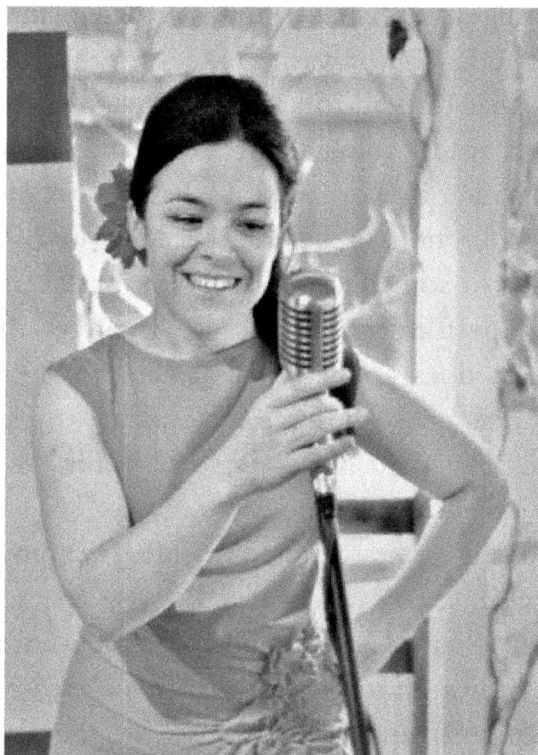

My Favorite Dance Partner

Jenny Hauser, Portland, Oregon, USA

At the time of our interview, I'd known Jenny in passing for several years—we had a number of mutual friends—but it wasn't until we sat down for this interview that I began to know her well. She shared her story with ready vulnerability and candidness in the backyard patio of a Portland café. Jenny's story is unique to this collection not just because it offers the perspective of someone who is both a blues dancer and a musical performer but because it offers that of a person who does not view all of her experiences with blues dancing as positive. Nonetheless, she also recognizes that dancing is responsible for "everything wonderful that my life is now."

"Dancing first entered my life when, toward the end of my marriage, I decided I was going to do the things that I loved and found joy in. I went back to musical theater and was cast in *South Pacific*. We were doing a performance to advertise for the show, and since it took place during a time period when there was swing dancing, we hired a couple of swing dancers for one of the scenes.

"After the performance, one of the dancers came up to me and asked me to dance. I told him I didn't know how to dance; it turns out he was a teacher, and he gave me his business card, which I kept in my wallet for a year. When my husband and I divorced, I decided that's what I was going to do for myself. I was going to start swing dancing because I enjoyed watching it so much."

Jenny had been married since she was sixteen years old. She recalled who she was when she left him after ten years of marriage. "I was pretty naïve to the ways of the world and pretty sheltered because my ex-husband was really controlling. I lived only twenty miles from Portland, but I had never driven in the city before, since my husband wouldn't let me do anything on my own. I remember trying to figure out how to get to dances; I was on the phone with my mom—this was before GPS—and she'd have to guide me to all these different places."

Jenny's mother helped her get to dances in another way too. She offered to babysit Jenny's ten-year-old daughter. "I'd come home from work and have dinner with my daughter, and then she'd go to bed and I'd go out dancing. It was the first time as an adult I was able to be myself without having a title of 'mom' or 'wife.' So it was really freeing to go into the city and go out dancing by myself." Jenny quickly became "completely addicted" to swing dancing, through which she was also introduced to blues. She thoroughly enjoyed the artistry of blues dancing but wasn't as comfortable with the intimacy.

Having experienced sexual intimacy with only one man, she found that the close connection adherent to blues was an experience she both appreciated and feared. "When I'm dancing with someone I'm comfortable with, I'm able to experience moments of intimacy in a very controlled, timed-out way—for just a three-minute song. I don't have to worry about giving more than that. But I have a lot of reservations about blues dancing because I've felt like at times people were taking things that I'm not willing to give.

"It might be a hang-up that I have, because ever since puberty I've been taken advantage of by men. People tell me the men there aren't really behaving that way—and if they are, then I need to set boundaries—but I'm still trying to figure out if it's just a figment of my own insecurities or if it's reality and justified that I feel that way."

It is because of that reason Jenny doesn't dance partnered blues very often. However, she has found another way to satisfy her love of the music and dance. She understood that it wasn't so much the physical connection with others that she loved about dancing—it was simply dancing. And, it turned out, performing.

"My whole world changed after I started dancing. I didn't realize that seven years later I'd still be involved in the dance scene. From swing dancing, I started blues dancing, and then I started singing swing and jump blues with the band 12th Avenue Hot Club and dancing for the blues band the Strange Tones. I don't mind singing or performing for blues dancers because there's a distance between the musicians on stage and the dancers on the floor; there's still an exchange that happens in the energy of the room, but it's one that feels safe for me."

Even though Jenny has her personal reservations about blues dancing, she enjoys exposing others to another perspective—including local blues musicians themselves. "I think some musicians feel blues dancers are a weird subculture of people who just grind with each other to their music. So I get the opportunity to explain the dance connection. They then get a little better understanding of it."

Jenny, in turn, has received the gift of exposure to new music and friendships through her relationship with local bands. "Dancing opened me up to all kinds of blues music; I grew up listening to swing and jump blues, but now I'm aware of a whole other realm of jazz and blues. And I got to develop friendships with the Strange Tones and other local well known musicians, which was really unexpected. They're some of my best friends now."

The contributions that blues music and dancing have made to Jenny's life don't stop there; lessons from the dance floor have helped her become strong in who she is. "Dancing definitely taught me not to take myself seriously. I've learned not to worry about how someone else perceives my dancing. It doesn't matter if people think I'm a good dancer—I just want to have fun dancing. By making that choice, you can be freer with how you dance and how comfortable you are taking risks. It's definitely symbiotic with just being okay with yourself in general—it puts that into dance form."

This shift was a major turning point for Jenny; as an adolescent and as a young adult, she didn't feel she fit in anywhere. As a teenage mother, she had a lot of barriers to break through with all social groups she encountered. "I didn't fit in with my peers because I was a mom, and I didn't fit in with other mothers who had children my daughter's age. Just going to parent meetings or to volunteer in the classroom was extremely awkward; I wasn't able to connect with others, or they didn't want to connect with me. So when I went out into the dance community, I just went, 'This is who I am.' I was really open, really honest. I stopped worrying about judgment, because judgment was already such a part of my everyday life."

That is a lesson she hopes may one day carry over into her daughter's life. I asked her what her daughter thought of her dancing, and she was quick to reply, "My daughter is pretty insightful; she has been able to recognize how happy dancing makes me. I wish we could share it together, but she doesn't show any interest in dancing." Jenny reflected momentarily, as if considering something for the first time. "But I hope she does one day. I hope she does because it breaks down a lot of personal barriers to be that open in front of all those people."

At this point, the sky began to turn gray, and a light rain began to fall, prompting me to ask for any final remarks as to what the blues had offered her life. Jenny said thoughtfully, "You know, I hope that I marry somebody who dances. I hope I find somebody who wants to dance with me forever. I went on this cruise once, and there was this couple dancing every dance together. They had been dancing together since they were in their twenties, and they are now in their eighties. They were just so great to watch; I knew they could bust a move and cut a rug at one point, and now they're totally stiff, and they can't move much, but it brings them joy to do it, and it lifts people up to watch. So I hope it's something that I can carry with me for the rest of my life."

Jenny shook her head and revised part of her statement—she knew she didn't need anyone but herself in order to carry dance with her forever. "Actually, I feel a connection more from the music than I do a dance partner. I even have dance parties by myself. I'll put on Dinah Washington, and I'll just have a dance party in my living room. And in that moment, I feel euphoric—like when you have a partner you really connect with. The fact that I can have that on my own...I guess...maybe I'm my favorite dance partner."

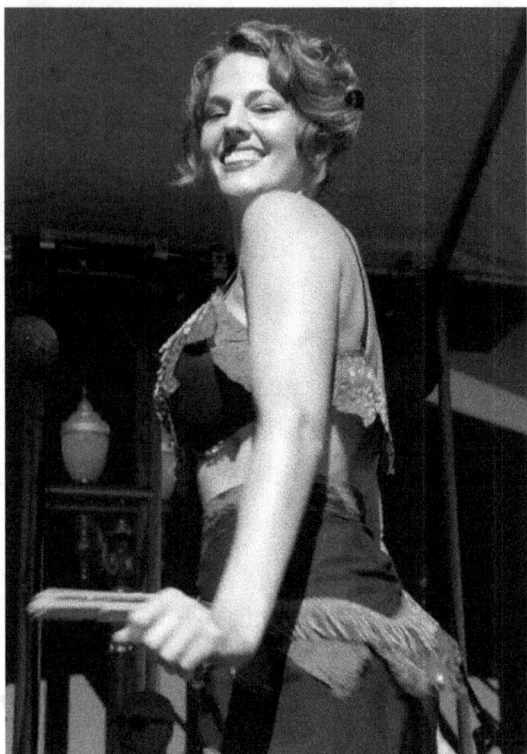

Music Is the Third Person in the Dance

Dean Mueller, Portland, Oregon, USA

Dean was one of the first blues dancers I met in Portland, at what was known as the Tango House—a private residence converted into a dance studio and occasionally rented out as a venue for dance parties. I was new to the city; the weekly blues dance was my introduction to a social community in Portland. And I was new to blues dancing. As it turned out, so was Dean.

"I have no idea what I'm doing, but would you like to dance with me?" Dean's first words to me were something to that effect. I sighed in great relief, as that meant I was not the only one who had no idea what to do. We figured it out together. We also ended up uncovering our mutual love of live music; Dean shared that he played bass in a West Coast blues band, and I enthusiastically divulged that I had worked at a renowned music venue in Nashville. His reaction filled me with joy—he knew the venue. At a time when I was feeling nostalgic for what I'd left behind in Nashville— from the music scene to the dance friends I'd made there—it felt good to be able to talk with someone who recognized some of the locations I associated with home.

Although we were both relatively new to blues dancing, I remember our dance connection being strong. He became one of the dancers I sought out each week. That was over eight years ago; we still run into each other at dances but not nearly as often. Instead, we're more likely to see each other at a live music event—usually one at which he's performing. He amazes many in the audience by his ability to play bass on stage, then step down for a few partner dances before resuming his position with the band.

When not dancing together, our communication almost always centers on music—which is why I never knew much about his personal story, until we sat down for this interview. What I found fascinating was that it was a physical ailment that led Dean to pursue a career in music. His job required heavy computer work, which caused him to develop severe repetitive strain energies with his left hand, forearm, and shoulder. He had set aside music to focus on his work, but the injury brought his awareness to how much music meant to him.

"I realized how fragile the body can be; I always wanted to get back to playing bass, and I just kept putting it off. Now all of a sudden I was having this serious problem with my hand and arm, wondering if I'd be able to play at all."

Dean could hardly turn a doorknob at the time, but he found he could play bass. "Playing the upright is really intense—which, as it turns out, was probably the best thing for me. I went for two years with all that pain, but when I started playing a lot in 2004, my problems just started going away. I think it's a combination of doing what you love doing and the fact that muscular-wise I was doing something so completely different; I was actually strengthening myself in ways I needed."

Dean began to take a career in music seriously. "I enrolled in Portland Community College's professional music program. I started studying engineering and sight singing and just started playing a lot." A significant turning point was when he went to Port Townsend, Washington, to attend jazz and acoustic blues workshops. The jazz workshop week didn't speak to him so much, but his experience at the blues week was different. "It just felt so good; it was such a relaxing experience compared to the previous week. I fell right into the blues group there. I met a lot of legendary blues musicians who are no longer with us—Honey Boy Edwards, Louisiana Red, John Cephas. When the weekend came, several of them asked me to play at the big show, so I did about four gigs in front of a couple thousand people. After that weekend, I thought, 'Okay, I'm going to go back home, and I'm going to be a blues musician. It just felt so good; I felt I'd proven to myself that I could do it."

The workshop not only provided an affirmation that he could make a career out of music but nurtured Dean's love for acoustic blues music. "I'd always been tied into rock-oriented blues when I was growing up, like Led Zeppelin—the bass player John Paul Jones was really rooted in blues—and Eric Clapton, Cream, and the Allman Brothers. The older stuff really didn't touch me until I went to the blues workshop, and I got to play with those guys. Sitting next to someone playing the real deal—not through a recording—and having to just join in and play without knowing the music, and having that feeling that takes over your whole body when it's really working…that's how I started to really love stripped down versions of blues music."

It's no wonder Dean felt a connection to blues music. He grew up in Chicago, a hotbed for both traditional and contemporary blues. "I saw Stevie Ray Vaughn many times before he died, but I didn't know old-school Chicago blues that much. I did see Willie Dixon—that was amazing—but even he was doing the modern, slicked-out version of his original songs. I loved that genre of blues—I still like it, and I still listen to it, but I mostly listen to older stuff, 1950s and older now."

I asked Dean what it was about blues music that moved him so deeply. He offered, "Blues is very emotional music, it's not technical music generally. I think why I like older blues music is because it's closer to the emotion that generated it. You can change the music and make it more modern, but I think you have to retain the emotion. There's probably some rhythmic music in various countries that is very emotional too, that creates those vibrations in your body, but to me the real deal is blues music."

Back in Portland, conveniently another hotbed for blues music, he sought out blues jams and other networking opportunities within the blues community. "I started going to blues jams at Duff's Garage. That was where I started to understand what the role of the bass is and get more experienced with West Coast blues. It was a really great jam; they were really welcoming to me when I was just learning. It was trial by fire right up there on stage, and it was really great."

Through the connections he made at the blues jam, Dean was hired to play for three different blues bands, each with its own particular style—West Coast blues, Texas electric blues, and vintage blues. It was the West Coast blues band—the Insomniacs—that put Dean on the map. The band won a Muddy Award from Oregon's prestigious Cascade Blues Association for Best New Act of 2006 and another later for Best Contemporary Act of 2007. They were also nominated for a 2008 Best New Artist Debut Award from the Blues Foundation in Memphis.

Fans began to take notice—not just with their ears but with their feet. It's hard to listen to the Insomniacs and not be compelled to dance. Dean witnessed that particular audience reaction and saw an opportunity. "At the time of the band's initial success, I had pretty much taken over all the booking and promotion. It was a great band with great music, but it became a question of how do you get it out to people? That's when I got involved with the dance scene.

"I saw a group of swing dancers at Duff's Garage, and I asked one of them about their dancing. She told me about West Coast Swing and East Coast Swing and blues, and I decided I needed to figure how to get some of those people to our shows. I didn't dance at all; I was very self-conscious and didn't think I could do it. I was one of those musicians who got asked to dance all the time and always said no." Dean laughed, and I considered how far he had come—knowing that he is now a regular on the dance floor.

Dean was so determined to figure out how the dance community worked that he enrolled in dance classes himself. "I was terrified; I could do the lesson part, but then when the dance started, I did maybe one dance and then left because it was fairly intimidating.

"Over time I found the right people to dance with so that it was comfortable for me. It didn't matter that I didn't think I was good—I just kept working at it. Then I started putting up Insomniacs posters and getting up during the break and saying, 'Hey, everyone, you should go and see live music.' At that point, they weren't coming out in mass to any live events at all— just a few of the swing people did."

Dean's efforts paid off. "We got really good turnouts for our album release parties as a result of that direct outreach. The dancers were key to the Insomniacs having such a great following; it was really important to have that young dance energy added to the show."

To his surprise, dancing added to Dean's musical career in another way.

"Dancing has significantly affected me as a musician; it's taught me to really listen, to leave a lot of space, and to be expressive in the music. Also to notice the crowd. If we saw dancers there, we would change what we played. That's what you do when you play to any room. You ask yourself, 'What does this room need? Do we need energy? Do we need openness? Do we need slow or fast dance energy?' You see what works and then you go from there."

Beyond what Dean gained from dance as a musician, he uncovered numerous rewards in his personal life. "What's great about dancing is you can go almost anywhere and—just like being a blues musician where you can just sit down and play if you know the language—you can just walk in and start dancing. I'd never been to any social dances before, so I didn't realize you just start dancing with random people. There's something great and liberating about that; you start to learn how to connect with different people in a dance scenario—and I totally went toward blues dancing because I thought it was the most expressive."

Expression is what Dean looks for most in a dance style, and what's most important to him in bringing that element out is the music. "It's there as the third person in the dance, so I think both people have to be very in tune with the music. I dance based completely on the music, so if it's an expressive song or a sad song, I like to pause a lot while I'm dancing. That doesn't mean the music stops, but that it breathes."

Once he's connected to the music, he embraces the connection with his partner. "You can have this connection with somebody who is just a friend or a stranger who I may never see again. I'd never experienced that combining of chemistry before; you're touching them more than just physically. Playing music with somebody is the closest thing I can think of to that, or talking to someone if you're really on the right wavelength—but that's usually because you're enamored and falling in love. I experienced that you can get that feeling with dance, even when you're not."

However, being in love with your dance partner brings the dance connection to a whole new level, as Dean can attest. "The girl I'm with now is a really good dancer, so just being able to go out there and be with somebody who dances is a great way to share life. It's amazing. As amazing as it is to dance with people you don't know and have that connection, it's even better to dance with somebody you really have a connection with. Now, I couldn't imagine being with somebody that didn't dance."

In addition to using dance as an outlet for connection, he uses his experience as testament to what is possible for him. "I've learned to be less afraid to do something that I absolutely didn't think I could do. I had no interest in dancing before—the only reason I did it is because I wanted to figure out how to market to that scene. And now I can do that with anything I want; it just takes letting go of whatever is constraining you in your own mind and going and doing it. One thing that's hard for me right now is singing. It's another thing that I always thought I didn't do well, so I just didn't do it. Every once in a while I start thinking, 'Dean, you should really start singing; you should do background vocals.' So that's another thing I should try to look at in the same way and tell myself, 'You can do this; you're just stopping yourself.'"

Dean has learned to pay more attention to those voices in his head—and his body. When he recalls his life before blues music and dance took such a hold of him, he remembers feeling stifled by a different kind of hold. "If I didn't find blues music and dancing, my life wouldn't be nearly as good. I probably would have just stayed stuck in life where I was at the time, and in pain. It was blues that allowed my body to let go of whatever it was holding onto—which was basically the message to quit doing what I was doing and instead do what I loved."

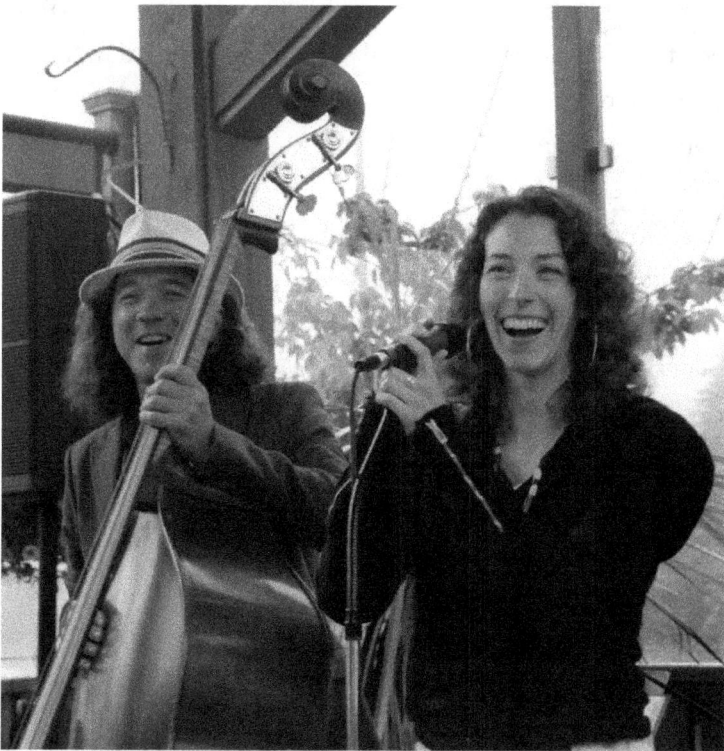

Photo by Renee Howard

Carrying the Blues Flag

Dan Nash, London, England

I had nearly resolved to include only five stories in this section; musicians with a connection to the blues dance community proved harder to track down than others. But then Dan Nash came to my attention. He played for a blues dance event in Europe recently and had told Brenda Russell, the event's organizer, "You know, a few years ago I was at one of the lowest points in my life; then I played for your blues dance camp, and everything turned around." The two continued to talk about the healing power of the music and dance, and the next day I received a message from Brenda: "You should interview Dan Nash."

Yes, I should, I agreed. But Dan proved hard to track down, with the eight-hour time difference and his busy gig schedule. We both were determined and made the interview happen early enough to be included in this collection.

Finally meeting him, over videocam, I realized I had seen Dan perform in London multiple times—at the European Blues Invasion dance event and at a small pub called the Joker. Whether he was playing for a large room of international dancers or a small room of chatty Brits—of varying degrees of inebriation—he gave his absolute all.

I felt the same in our interview. The book's topic is one that he feels passionate about; he has experienced both blues music and blues dance as transformational. Dan is not a dancer himself, but to play for a crowd that is engaged in his music to the degree that dancers are validates his role as a blues musician—a role which he'd come to define as our discussion went on.

As if to relax into the interview, Dan lit a cigarette and sat back comfortably on his couch. He tilted the video camera to center on his face and began. "There are only two things I've been passionate about in my life. One is blues; the other is Latin and Greek classical literature."

Already the interview was off in a direction I had not anticipated. I waited for him to continue.

"That's what I studied at university. At one time, I was sitting here wondering what those two things have in common, and I realized, fundamentally, they both strip everything back. When I'm talking about classics, by the way, I'm talking about Homeric poetry, which is an oral tradition because the people were suppressed from being able to write—they were illiterate due to lack of educational opportunities. It was very raw; it said it exactly how it was. And blues is the same—it comes from a suppressed community. Academically, that's what I found fascinating about blues, and why I locked myself away for over four years and learned to play it."

Dan was full of many surprises, I learned as the interview went on. He looks like a blues man—he wears a fedora or a newsboy hat, depending on the gig; facial scruff and a rough-around-the-edges but gentle grin. And he's also an accountant. Rather than contradict each other, he defends, these two roles keep him balanced. He declares he does not have the discipline to be able to manage his creative energy without time working in business.

And discipline must abound in his work—he is primarily a self-taught musician. He has not only poured over blues recordings to study the art but taken it upon himself to learn the history—from books and from the early blues musicians themselves. Part of his research took him to America for a six-week road trip. "I went to all the locations that I knew about through the books I'd read—where certain blues players were buried, where they were seen playing for the first time, and so on. I knocked on doors and asked, 'Who's the oldest guitarist in this town?' And you know, down South they'll tell you, and the guy will invite you in. I got to jam with legends and film them playing acoustic guitars. I interviewed Honey Boy Edwards, Robert Johnson's granddaughter, Muddy Waters's younger brother (Robert Morganfield), and contemporary artists in Louisiana." Dan dreams of being able to turn his research into a documentary someday, but for now the twenty-four hours of footage serve as a personal relic of having touched a bygone era.

Dan's initial exposure to blues music happened well before that 2007 road trip. His infatuation began when he was "too young to understand it." He compared his experience to that of recognizing a beautiful woman for the first time, before he knew what "fancying someone was."

He described the first time he heard early African American blues music, at thirteen years old: "I knew there was a transmission of someone's feeling, a digging deep into their soul, without being inhibited to deliver their performance with honesty."

It would be several years yet, however, before the blues would absorb his attention again. Although he dabbled in guitar—his whole family was musical, and "there were always guitars lying around"—his real commitment to blues music began after a visit to Tennessee as an adult. His dad had moved there from England after marrying an American woman. "Me and my dad were best buddies, so I told him I'd be happy come visit and hang out with him and the new missus, but I wanted three days of just me and him on the road."

In addition to exploring Nashville, the two visited Memphis. "That's when I saw the blues players out there and heard a live harmonica through the microphone. I hadn't played guitar properly for a while, but when I heard them play, I got really into it." He recalled going to a guitar shop in Nashville and picking up some instructional DVDs. "I figured I could teach myself. I bought some music of Muddy Waters and Robert Johnson; when I brought them to the counter, the guy looked at the Robert Johnson one and laughed and said, 'This guy plays bass, rhythm, and lead—all at the same time. That's impossible.'" Dan nodded and grinned, knowing he wanted to embark on a journey that sounded so hard core.

"For the next four years, I barely left home after work. I'd come home and play for four or five hours, listening to everything I possibly could. I loved it—the music and the subject. The background of it really touched a nerve in me." Dan knew almost from the start, however, that his passion would never prove lucrative. "When I went to see Muddy Waters's grave and saw that it was about the size of my thumbnail, I thought that if he isn't going to make a fortune out of playing the blues, nobody is. But I love it enough to accept that I'll never be able to make a living off of it."

It's just as well, he concluded, as there is a risk involved. "It's important to continue to love your art for the same reason you started loving it in the first place; it's very dangerous to drop everything and do it for a living—you can end up resenting the thing you loved."

Dan has other goals and rewards with his music. "My role as a musician is to carry the blues flag—to play it as authentically as I can without having been in that place in that period, to show people how it was. Which is the beauty of the dance piece." Dan suddenly got excited, his arm raised to emphasize his next point.

"My study only ever came from a musician's point of view. In the beginning, jazz was made to be danced and be rowdy to; that gets lost on a record. I missed that point until I met the dancers and felt the reciprocal energy between the musicians and dancers. When I'm playing and I see someone's feet doing something, I might imitate it with my guitar; they hear me imitating it, so they do something else to see if I can do that. There's this bouncing, growing energy that creates the most amazing communal feeling."

Dan's introduction to the dance scene initially came through London's swing dance community—which at the time was also organizing the community's blues dance events. He wasn't aware of either scene until a musician friend turned him onto it. "I was working five days a week and had no time to seek out gigs. I asked my friend if he knew of any scenes going on, and he said, 'Funnily enough, I just did a gig for some dancers.' I was like 'What? People dance to blues?' He told me they do, just as you'd imagine it—close contact, one on one, usually late at night after fast stuff has been going on. He passed me his contact, and it snowballed from there."

Event organizers aren't always local—and of course a significant percentage of attendees are not local either. Therefore, when word gets out that there's a good band to dance to, other regional or international communities end up hiring them for their events. "I'd say probably two-thirds of what I make from playing music comes out of the dance community," he shared.

But the community is not just a source of income for Dan—it's a source of inspiration. The whole experience came as a surprise to him. "I remember I didn't know what to expect. When I first started playing, my initial feeling was 'I've got to be on my game' because you could hear a pin drop in there; it's not like being in a pub, where if you screw up a couple of notes, no one hears it—they're all talking and drinking. At the dance event, I was actually being listened to. If you decide to make one little change in the rhythm, then you're going to see that whole change across the floor."

That experience was transformative for Dan, not just in regards to his career. "As far as other personal issues were concerned, I was probably at the peak of badness. I remember thinking, 'These guys are all high, and they're all clean. What is this secret about?' I could imagine that kind of experience in a small town where everyone knows each other, but when you live in a really busy city like London and there's all this love in one room with no agenda whatsoever—and no fake high—I realized, 'These people are good for me. Being with these people is good for me.' I left that gig thinking, '*Ahhh*. Life isn't so bad.'"

Dan's involvement with the dance community grew from there, along with the pleasure he experiences at his gigs. "I now know what it's like for people who enjoy their jobs; I have a taste of it when I do this. When I go to work a dance camp or festival in Europe, where I'm surrounded by these lovely people, I feel like it's the best therapy that a human being can have. I'm receiving love from loads of directions without even reaching out for it."

And he gets to play what he loves the most. "I remember reading a quote by Bob Margolin—Muddy Waters's guitarist— that if Muddy could have only played slow blues, he would have. The only reason he played fast blues is because that's what his audience wanted. I feel exactly the same; to be able to deliver deep feeling, you need space. You need slow blues.

"When I play clubs and bars, the comments are 'Don't you know any faster stuff?' With blues dancers, it's the opposite. I don't have to worry about having to do a fast song if I've just done a couple of slow songs."

When Dan is on stage performing, there's something else he doesn't have to worry about either—feeling vulnerable. He doesn't write his own music for that reason. "To be able to write, you've got to be honest and truthful and dig deep, and the Englishman in me finds it very difficult to share the deepest and darkest part of myself with an audience. When I'm singing someone else's songs, I am sharing that part of myself with the audience, but I don't feel as vulnerable."

Dan paused for a moment before continuing his thought. "There's a line you have to cross from an emotional perspective where you're prepared to look an audience in the eye and deliver something that's coming from your heart rather than Robert Johnson's or Muddy Waters's heart." Dan winked and added with a sly smile, "So they think."

Dan still admits that "maybe someday" he will feel called to write his own songs. "For years I told myself that eventually I'd be inspired to write; I wrote every single song for the first band I was in when I was fourteen and wasn't inhibited—and they were good for my age. I've never written a thing since, but I've stopped waiting around for the inspiration to come because I don't think that's what my role is within the blues community.

"My job as a musician is to deliver a feeling with as much authenticity as I can and to share how wonderful this music is. It's like the feeling of being in church and singing with loads of people; if you're in that moment, you don't need to turn to each other and say, 'Isn't this wonderful?' And that's what I'm trying to do with blues—I'm trying to say, 'Isn't this wonderful?' without actually stopping and pointing it out."

Therefore, Dan sees himself less as an innovator and more as a messenger. "I have chosen a specific era of blues to specialize in. I feel aggrieved that I never got to see anyone in concert—apart from B. B. King—from the generation and the area I consider to be so rich in talent, as well as cruelty and cotton" Dan paused long enough for me to notice the poetic nature of his words and sense his songwriting potential. "I'm very fussy about blues players worth watching; as far as I'm concerned, almost everyone who's good is dead."

A bold statement, but one that emphasizes the importance of not letting authentic reproduction of the original music die off. Of that he's not worried. "My thoughts are that for as long as human beings have hearts and souls—which will be till the day that we cease to exist—there will be people who will be passionate about blues. As with any art, it's cyclical; it falls in and out of favor with the public." Perhaps it is his nature as an accountant to notice an influential factor in that cycle. "A lot of that has to do with social circumstances;

I noticed when the credit crunch came, my gigs increased twofold because people could suddenly relate."

Dan doesn't see his role as that of a dancer, either. At least not of blues. "If someone puts a funk record on, man, I'm on the floor, but with blues dancing, there are only certain members of the dance community—who I am friends with—I can dance with and not feel inhibited."

Aside from that fact, he admits, "I'm not much of a team player. That's why if you ever see me play with a band, it's basically my solo set with the band." Dan explained that he prefers to focus on other aspects of relationship and communication. He picked up his guitar and said, "Like the one between me and my baby, who I'm talking to all the time." He said it's different than a dance, however, because "she does exactly what I tell her to do when I tell her to do it—unlike a dance partner, where the compliance to will is mutual."

He has thought long and hard about it, and he realizes he actually plays a part in the latter two of three relationships at a dance. "There are three relationships going on: the relationship between a dancer and their partner, the relationship between the guitarist's voice and his guitar, and the relationship between the musician and the dancers. When those three relationships are in harmony, it's heaven."

He needs his day job to balance out playing music, and he needs the relationship with his guitar to balance out all the strife inherent to the rest of life.

"Playing the blues is the only means by which I can *aaaarghhh.*" Dan raised his fist and gritted his teeth. "Some people want to hit a punching bag; some people want to go for a run. I want to get on stage for an hour and a half and show people how amazing this music is."

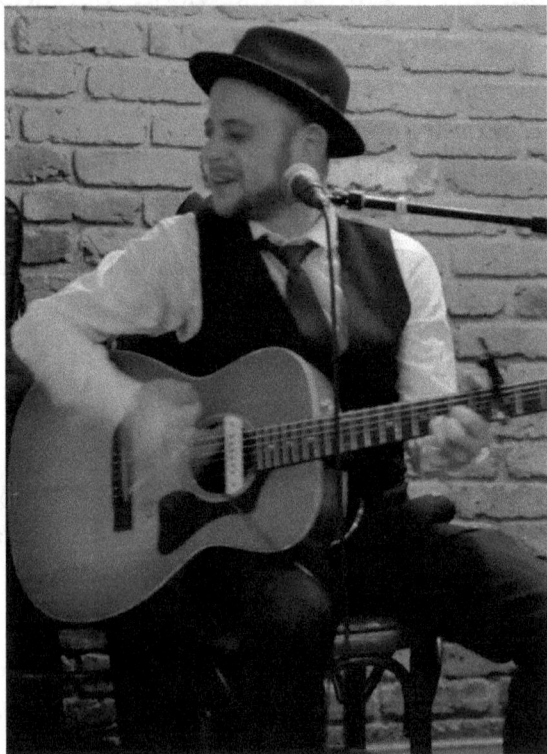

Photo by Antonio García Martín

I'll Remember This Night the Rest of My Life

Curtis Salgado, Portland, Oregon, USA

If it weren't for Curtis, this book might not exist. As described in the introduction, it was his performance at the 2013 Rose City Blues dance festival in Portland, Oregon, that led to a moment of inspiration. It was a night I'll always remember.

It was clear the night was a powerful one for him too; I'd seen him perform many times before, but I had not seen him react so emotionally at the end of his set, nor with such gratitude. He was grateful for the audience's awareness and appreciation of his music but even more so for our offering him hope that blues music had a chance. It might not die out with the last remaining members of the generation that had seen the original blues legends perform live.

A friend introduced me to Curtis after another of his performances, and I told him about this project. I didn't have to convince him to be a part of it; he wanted nothing more than to share his passion and perspective—one that emphasizes we know the history—with the blues dance community. It's a topic that gets Curtis riled up, for good reason.

"Blues dancers need to know the history. Where this music came from. I'm telling you, *everyone* should know the history. Is it going to make a difference if they do? Is it going to make them dance better? I doubt it.

No. But I just think it would be nice, because otherwise it's going to disappear."

I told him I wanted to share his message, but I needed more information. We agreed to meet for an interview a couple of weeks later. Since the interview would be recorded, I needed a relatively quiet place to meet. I picked a teahouse that was within the neighborhood we both lived in. The Tao of Tea had resided there as a thriving business for nearly twenty years; however, it was Curtis's inaugural visit.

We were the first customers of the day; I wondered how the sweet, pixie-like waitress may have perceived our joint arrival. He walked in slowly, his neck twisting this way and that as his eyes took in the wall of cascading water, the rock formations, and the wooden and bamboo furniture. The ambience was tranquil, the music classical Chinese, and I suddenly wondered if I had chosen the right place. As if reading my mind, he began to nod and said, "I like it. I should bring my girlfriend here."

I sighed in relief. I would have another scare, however, when we sat down and he saw the menu. Nearly twenty pages of tea options. "You're going to need to help me with this," he began. I told him I was happy to. He paused before adding, "You know, the Beatles were into this stuff." He started warming up to the idea of tea over coffee, or any other beverage.

At that point, the waitress returned and offered him the help he needed. "Do you have any questions?" she asked.

"Yes, I need something for my stomach."

She looked at him warmly and asked, like a patient nurse, "What is the issue you have with your stomach?"

"It's upset. I went to the casino last night and ate something I shouldn't have. I was up all night."

She referred him to the herbal infusions section of the menu, and the one that promised to taste of licorice sold him.

I asked him if he could recall his earliest exposure to blues music. His memories of blues were mixed with jazz—genres he considers almost one and the same—and like himself, were birthed through his parents. "My parents grew up in the swing era; they were born around 1918, so by the time they were teenagers, the music that came through their lives was jazz. When I was growing up, they had these old records; they'd play Count Basie, Fats Waller, Ray Charles, and boogie-woogie piano players. That music would hit my audio nerve, and you know, you start to listen to that stuff and pretty soon you become attached to it. One of the biggest albums that blew me away was Benny Goodman's *Live at Carnegie Hall*."

At this point, the waitress came back with our tea. He tried a sip of his and was pleased. My tea caught his attention more, however. The flowers floating around intrigued him, and he asked, "Do you mind if I try some of that?" I offered him a sip, and his face relaxed. "That's fantastic." I smiled at his delight, and he continued.

"So, on the back of these records were descriptions written by music critics and liner notes. Those liner notes, they'd put me onto things. There was a song where they're jamming, and then it breaks into piano and this whole other approach; that struck me, and I read more about it in the liner notes. I'll never forget that."

When he was thirteen years old, Curtis had the opportunity to see Count Basie live, at the University of Oregon's basketball arena in Eugene, where he grew up. "It was an all-black big band; I was like, *wow*. The finest jazz musicians were on stage. I was hooked. I can still picture it. It changed my life. I remember saying, 'I want to do that!'"

Curtis initially worked toward his dream by taking guitar lessons, but his lessons didn't last long. "I had a mean guitar teacher who kicked me if I didn't hit the right note. The other reason I quit is because I didn't want to learn the technical side of music—how to read and how to practice my scales. I had a very good ear; I could hear something and then play it."

The technical side of music never impressed him much, which is why he gravitated toward blues rather than jazz. But Curtis will tell you that within jazz music, you can find the blues—in the form of a feeling. "The blues is a feeling. It's something you can hear and pinpoint in the music. Miles Davis is a blues player; he has all this technical ability, but he plays blues—you can hear it. And the same with Charlie Parker. You hear the blues in Billie Holiday; you hear the blues in Dinah

Washington. What they sing is just more technical or sophisticated, for lack of a better term."

Curtis credits that "mean guitar teacher" with leading him away from jazz and his mother for leading him to blues. "My mom brought me home a harmonica book called *How to Play Blues Harmonica.* For probably thirty years, it was the only harmonica book that existed on how to play blues.

"At that time, my older sister and brother were starting to buy blues records—this was the '60s, when folk music was coming in, and a lot of the folk-era movements were also discovering black blues masters who had recorded forty years earlier and were still alive. They started putting these guys on the college circuit, and with that, record companies started making these old songs available—Robert Johnson, Muddy Waters, Little Walter, Lightning Hopkins—all these collectors started going out and buying them, along with young college kids. And I was one of them."

A couple albums in particular inspired Curtis to continue with his harmonica study—and his dedication to blues performance. His brother passed him a Paul Butterfield record that blew him away. Who was this "twentysomething-year-old white kid playing the shit out of harmonica?" he asked himself. He was incredulous. Once again, he turned to the liner notes.

The song that most struck him was written by W. Jacobs. Further research revealed that was Little Walter—so he got his hands on one of his albums. "Once I heard Little Walter, that was it. It changed everything. It was the deepest low-down blues and the nastiest harmonica playing." He'd never felt more inspired to play.

Of course, Curtis didn't just play harmonica. He was an extremely talented singer; a trait his kindergarten teacher made sure others took note of. "In kindergarten, a teacher pinned a note on my chest. This teacher, I can still see her in my mind's eye, she says, 'Make sure your mother gets this.' So when I get home, my mother reads it and says, 'Your teachers says you can sing—that you have a nice voice and that you're going to learn these songs.'"

Luckily for Curtis, his mother was a piano player, and she immediately set about teaching her son the two songs the teacher requested: "I've Been Working on the Railroad" and "Jesus Loves Me." "One day at school we went to the auditorium, and we practiced it. I didn't make any connection that I had been rehearsing for an assembly—I was just doing as I was told—but one day all our parents were there in the auditorium.

"So I'm up on stage along with this other little boy next to me—the two of us are to sing together. So I start singing 'Jesus Loves Me,' while he stays stiff as a board. I can still see him in my mind, I remember looking up at him—he was taller than me—and I'm going, 'Jesus loves me, this I know...,' and he's not singing at all. So I continue, 'Cuz the BIBLE'—I poked him with my elbow—'tells me so...,' and the audience starts laughing. I went on, 'Little ones to HIM belong'—another jab, more laughing. And he just stood solid with stage fright while I sang both songs by myself. I was hooked because the audience adored me. I knew I had won the day."

He played his first professional gig at sixteen and by eighteen was a known name in his local community's bar scene. When Curtis joined forces with others to form the Nighthawks, he gained popularity throughout the Pacific Northwest.

Things really started to take off when, in 1973, he met Robert Cray. The two became friends and began jamming together and sitting in with each other's bands. A few years later, he gained additional notoriety when comedian and actor John Belushi was in Eugene filming *Animal House*. Belushi was fortunate enough to catch one of Curtis's performances. Another friendship ensued, and partially due to Curtis's having taught John about blues music and history, the idea for the motion picture *The Blues Brothers* was born. The record album released in collaboration with the film, *Briefcase Full of Blues*, is dedicated to Curtis.

The more exposed Curtis got to the national blues community, the more he realized he had outgrown his own band. It was then that he was invited to join the more dynamic Robert Cray Band, which quickly grew in prestige. Curtis got to share stages with blues legends such as Muddy Waters, Bobby Bland, and Bonnie Raitt. When he parted ways with the Robert Cray Band in 1982, he formed his own band—Curtis Salgado & the Stilettos. He released his first solo album a decade later and began touring the country, forming a strong following. He would later go on to tour and sing with Santana and Steve Miller.

As Curtis was telling me about how it felt to share the stage with such legends, the waitress returned to check on us. "How's the tea?" she asked Curtis. He replied sincerely, with a hint of humor, "Perfect. I'm healing," before continuing his story without missing a beat.

"I mean, Muddy Waters! Muddy changed the course of music, and I was in a room with him, let alone playing and singing with him? I got to play with all those guys. It's just mind-blowing."

Curtis paused for a moment before bringing us back to the initial, critical point he wanted to make to readers of this book.

"That's why I think it's important that the blues dance community knows the history. I think they would enjoy their dancing better. The idea of two bodies connecting and moving together—it's very beautiful, but you know what? This music isn't just blues. It's also bluegrass and roots and Irish music; it's Scottish music and mountain music and the mixture of all of those. It's like if you're a chef, you have all these ingredients sitting out there; you have Spanish ingredients, French ingredients, Caribbean, African, all these things—that is what America is. That is why this music is so special, because it's all those things in a gumbo. That's what brings out a more exotic, sexy flavor—those African and Caribbean spices in there; throw in some cayenne red pepper, and now things start to get syncopated. Blues is the whole world blended."

I asked Curtis if Rose City Blues was his first exposure to the contemporary blues dance scene; it was certainly his first time playing a show specifically for dancers, but he'd noticed blues dancers before, without knowing about the existence of the scene. The first dancer he saw was, interestingly, a fellow musician friend—Dean Mueller.

To listen to Curtis share his reaction had me in stitches. "I was at a bar and Dean starts dancing with this woman. He's doing this smooth, sexy thing, and I thought, 'Who's *that*? She's fine! This dude is such a player—I didn't know that!' Then he starts dancing with another girl, and *she's* fine, and then *another* one...I'm like, '*Three* of them?!' I went up to him and said, 'Dude, you *rock*! What are you, a pimp or something?' And he goes, 'No, I do blues dancing.' So that was when I first heard of it."

Curtis's second exposure to a blues dancer was at one of his shows; he'd noticed Brenda Russell solo dancing toward the front of the stage for the entire duration of his gig. At the end of the set, he leaned over and asked her, "Who are you? You're a great dancer!" "And she says her name and tells me I was going to be playing at one of the dance community's events. I said, 'That's cool...I am?!' It didn't really sink in."

Since booking for Curtis's shows was done through his booking agent, he was not always aware of the particulars of each gig. As it turned out, no one had succeeded in telling him what kind of music blues dancers dance to. Curtis had just released an R&B album, and his shows were focused on promoting that style of up-tempo funk and soul music. When he learned—just before the gig—that blues dancers only dance to slow- or moderate-tempo tunes, he panicked.

"I only play one slow song per show. I love playing slow blues, but in my experience, an audience wants to pop! So I thought, 'Aww, man, what am I going to do?!' So I go to the venue, and I tell my band, 'Listen, you guys, we can't play our show. Our show goes *bang bang bang,* and we can't play that. We're going to have to jam blues, or they're going to laugh us out of this house and never have us back.'"

Kevin Selfe—whose story is earlier in this section— was at the show, and Curtis approached him to discuss his predicament. Kevin invited him upstairs, where a smaller studio was playing deejayed music for a group of blues dancers. "This is what they dance to," he told him.

Curtis's reaction was distinct. "We walk in this room, and the deejay is playing 'Nineteen Years Old,' by Muddy Waters—the *original* low-down, rotten, recorded-in-1949 version—and there's twenty-five youngsters in there dancing to it, all dressed to the nines, right out of the '30s. I thought I was in heaven!

"It was not my typical audience—everyone was half my age or younger, and that was refreshing. Two things hit me—one is that there is hope that this music can stay alive. I don't know if this music will stay alive in terms of Muddy Waters or Howlin' Wolf, because they don't make 'em like that anymore. It's all been done, and you won't see it again. That's why the history is important to know...so you can hand your kid a Little Walter record. Maybe it will hit them like it hit me."

Curtis went back downstairs and took the stage with his band. He knew he had the first song ready—the one slow song he plays in his set is the opening song. His band kicked it off, and after the first few beats, he was amazed to see the dancers instantly respond with sheer joy—raising their arms and cheering. Curtis was in shock. "I don't have much hair, but if I did, it would have all been standing up straight. I was like, 'What?! No one does that!!' It was wonderful. So then I turned around to the band and said, 'Okay, I want you to do this, and you to do this.' So we played another slow song, and everyone danced to it...very happily—at the end the dancers went, 'Yay!' So I just kept thinking of slow songs. We played slow blues all night with my band, which had never done that before. My drummer thought it was boring. *I* loved it."

The show hit its peak toward the end of the night; Curtis launched into "Hoochie Coochie Man"—a Muddy Waters song—causing the dancers to turn from their partners and come to the stage. "I held this long note—that got people to start listening; I held it indefinitely, and the audience went wild. When the song ended in its entirety, I looked down, and there were *roses* at my feet. I was like, *wow*. When you're in a room with people who are half my age who are picking up on what

I'm throwing down—who *get* it—that made me extremely happy. I was stunned. It gave me hope. It was one of the best experiences I've ever had. I will remember that night the rest of my life."

Curtis's euphoria did weaken slightly, however, when he learned after the show that a lot of the dancers in the community don't know the history behind what they dance to. That fact accentuated his fear that awareness of the historical importance of blues music could fade with his generation. "I've been in the business a long time. I'm *extremely* passionate. I love roots music, and I love the history of music. That's my life. So to play this music my whole life and then watch it disappear..." Curtis's voice trailed off, perhaps imagining how different his life would have been without blues.

His suggestion to young dancers is to do what he did. "I learned the history of the world through music. Reading and researching. 'Why this? Who invented that? Where's this come from?' Know the history. Listen to the lyrics and learn where it comes from. If it's moving you, you should know its history. Why is it moving you? What's behind this?"

Clearly, Curtis is passionate about learning musical history—but not in an archeological manner. "Don't study the blues from the perspective of 'He traveled here, and they came down and migrated...' As if talking about a dinosaur. Life just isn't like that. Don't try to make sense of it all. There is no *definition* of blues music—or blues dancing. It's however it makes you move.

"When you're dancing to blues, you have music you're listening to and steps that you're doing, but somebody's creating something new. There can be nobody saying that what you're doing isn't blues dancing. If someone says, 'That's not blues dancing,' just tell him, 'Different streaks for different freaks. That's great for you. This is blues dancing to me.' Music is in the ear of the beholder. Who's to say what is or what isn't in *any* situation? If you had a rule in blues music, tell that to John Lee Hooker. He just went with what he felt. The blues is a feeling. There are no rules."

Curtis had one other piece of advice he wants to distill to blues dancers. "What I noticed—what I loved—is that you dancers are keeping time in your head, with no bass or backbeat. That's *really* good for you. When there's only two people playing, a singer and a guitar and a harmonica, where is the pulse? It's in the guitar, and it's in your head, so you're making the very most out of the limited amount of what's happening.

"A great practice is to try dancing without music. Maybe give thirty seconds of a groove, and then turn the music off and continue dancing to it, keeping the beat in your head. Or play the song once all the way through and then take the music out. You'll learn to keep time. Time in music is it, it's the pocket."

At this point, we had been talking for over two hours. I wanted to respect his time—he had a gig to prepare for that night. But I had one more question. It was obvious to me that blues music had been transformational to Curtis's life in many ways, but I considered there may be additional elements of healing below the surface. And there were—literally. Curtis lifted his shirt to show me a broad scar stretching across his abdomen.

"It's a liver transplant. I'd been playing music all my life and had no health insurance. So musician friends of mine held a benefit. It had Steve Miller, Taj Mahal, Robert Cray, Everclear, Little Charlie and the Nightcats, and myself. We split the Rose Garden Arena in half and filled it up with like five thousand people. Everything was donated to me—the building, over three hundred volunteers; the *Oregonian* put two full-page ads in the newspaper; Kink radio pushed it; and we had the most incredible concert with this oddball mixture of people. We raised the money we thought we needed, and then at the last minute, the hospital said we needed $100,000 more in order to do the transplant. So two more people stepped up and gave me their life savings.

"How has blues music healed me? I owe the universe. How do you pay that back? I can't keep a straight face. I am *so* blessed."

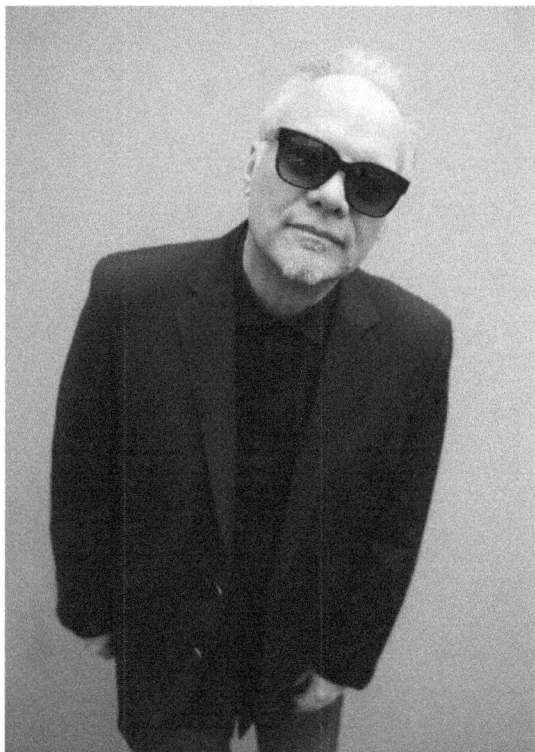
Photo by Jessica Keaveny

AUTHOR'S NOTE

Thank you for taking this journey with me—and with the thirty-six courageous story contributors. I hope this book has left you feeling inspired in numerous ways. If so, please share it with others—you never know who might embark on their own journey of transformation as a result.

So, what's my story, some of you may be wondering. Like all of our stories, my blues dance story is constantly evolving. A few years ago, I would have told you it's a story about finding the confidence to be comfortable moving my body and expressing my femininity. But that's a story I've already written about in my previous book, *Finding Ecstasy*.

These days, I would say my blues dance story is one about falling truly, deeply in love for the first time in my life—not just with the music or the movement but with a man I met on the blues dance floor. That man is responsible for leading me to break the social etiquette rule—and my own rule—of no making out on the dance floor. Sometimes we have to seize the moment, etiquette be damned.

And my blues dance story is also about this project. Layering other people's journeys with mine has led me to deeper self-reflection and understanding of the bigger picture. I already knew blues music and dancing were healing—that was obvious from my personal experience. But until this project, I had no idea just *how* healing—or just how many levels of transformation were taking place within my dance partners and those dancers all across the room and the globe. This book has allowed me the sacred opportunity to sit down one-on-one with people I had never met before and those I had danced with many times in the past and gain access to their souls.

Which is why the topic of transformation fascinates me so much; it's a topic that requires vulnerability. Those featured in this book have crossed over from the "dark side"—whatever that looked like for them—and are in a position to share what might work with those still struggling. Transformation isn't as much a subject of personal triumph as it is one of inspiration. It announces, "If I did it, so can you."

For many contributors to this book, they have agreed to enter into that vulnerable space in order to make that announcement—not only to me but to everyone who reads this book.

Because of that courage, I have met the most fascinating people, whom I may not have met otherwise. I have been blessed with the opportunity to sit down with musical performers I may have been too shy to approach without this particular purpose. I have learned so much about the history of this music and this dance that I love. All of that has now been added to my evolving blues journey.

I hope it's a journey that never ends.

ABOUT THE AUTHOR

Rebecca Pillsbury fell in love with stories as a precocious eight-year-old, building stacks of books taller than herself to take home from the library. She began writing her own stories soon after, entering writing contests and dreaming of being a published author as an adult.

Her first published book, *Finding Ecstasy*, was a prize winner in Christine Kloser's Transformational Author Writing Contest. She subsequently launched her own publishing company, Duende Press, through which she helps people such as business leaders, adventure travelers, and celebrities tell their transformational stories.

Rebecca currently resides in Portland, Oregon, though you may not find her there year-round—a vagabond spirit cannot be tamed. You can keep in touch with her at www.duendepressbooks.com—she loves to hear from readers!

DANCE RESOURCES

Visit this site for bonus material:
www.duendepressbooks.com/blues-bonus

Blues Dance Instruction

The instructors listed below teach in their local communities but also spend considerable time traveling the globe teaching at dance workshops and events.

Dave Madison (www.bluesdance.com)
Brenda Russell (www.brendadances.com)
Vicci Moore & Adamo Ciarallo
(www.adamoandvicci.com)
Andrew Sutton (www.danceninjas.com)
Velody (www.velody.co.uk)
Andrew Smith (www.andrewsmithdance.com)
Justin Riley (www.bluesrecess.com)

Blues Dance Events

This portal is managed by Drew Tronvig, and is a comprehensive resource for local and worldwide blues dance communities and events, and other blues dance resources such as videos, set-lists, and links to blues dance social media sites.

www.panadance.com

This calendar is managed by Dave Madison, and is a resource for worldwide blues dance workshops and exchanges, as well as other vintage dances such as Lindy Hop and balboa.

www.bluescal.com

Blues Dance Photography

My sincere gratitude to the following photographers for their contributions to this book.

Fredrik Lindbom (www.flfoto.se)
Evrim Icoz (www.evrimgallery.com)
Kai Liesirova
Patrick Fulgencio (www.patrickfulgencio.com)
Drew Tronvig (www.panadance.com)
Jason Roseweir
(www.roseweirphotography.co.uk)
Alexey Tolstoguzov
mswheelerphotography
Yugandhar Beesetty
Fabio Bortot (www.fabiobortot.com)
Samuel Nesbitt (www.samuelnesbitt.com)
John Krieger-Joven
Nuria Aguade (www.nuriaaguade.com)
Renee Howard
Eric Frommer
(www.ericfrommerphotography.com)
Sara White
Jessica Keaveny (www.jessicakeaveny.com)

Antonio García Martín
(www.antoniogarciamartin.com)
Alexandre Swidaneel (www.lightexmachina.com)
Bobby Bonsey (www.bbonsey.com)
Shane Meyers (www.speakeasy.photos)
Pete Gowing
Benoit Guerin
(www.facebook.com/benoitguerinphotography)
Jelena Lihhatsova
(www.jelenalihhatsova.wordpress.com)
Kate Voronova

Dance Filmography

The video technicians below create corporate videos, but also have passion and experience in dance filmography.

Ian Burke (www.promovideo.co.uk)
Devon Cooke (www.storybubble.ca)

Blues Musicians

These musicians are featured within this book:

Curtis Salgado (www.curtissalgado.com)
Dan Nash (www.dannashblues.com)
Kevin Selfe (www.kevinselfe.com)
Dean Mueller with Julie Amici
(www.deanmueller.com, www.julieamici.com)
Velody (www.velody.co.uk)
Jenny Hauser (www.strangetones.com)

BLUES PLAYLIST

Damon Stone: *Smokestack Lightnin'*, Howlin' Wolf

Brenda Russell: *Blues Before Sunrise*, John Lee Hooker

Dave Madison: *Pussycat Moan*, Katie Webster

Nadja Gross: *To Build a Home*, The Cinematic Orchestra

Kenneth Shipp: *Take Out Your False Teeth Daddy*, Margie Day

Andrew Sutton: *New Orleans Bump*, Wynton Marsalis

Cara Bennett: *That's a Pretty Good Love*, Big Maybelle

Eros Salvatore: *Wolf Dance*, Ronnie Earl

Anna Takkula: *I Wish I Knew How It Would Feel to Be Free*, Nina Simone

Alyx LeBeau: *Blues 2.0*, Fruteland Jackson

Laura Gioia: *It Hurts Me Too*, Elmore James

Clara Pochettino: *New Year Blues*, Glenn Crytzer and His Syncopators

Ryan Limbaugh: *Call off the Search*, Josh Kumra

Robert Grandison: *Mannish Boy*, Muddy Waters

Kai Stiller: *The Thrill Is Gone*, B.B. King

Lorna: *Wade in the Water*, Eva Cassidy

Jana Jade: *Just Ask*, Lake Street Dive

Jenny Lynn: *My Daddy Rocks Me*, Marty Grosz

Krunal Waghela: *Slow Train*, Joe Bonamassa

Stella: *Sittin' on Top of the World*, Ray Charles

Surahbhi McMellahn: *I Feel Blue*, Alif Tree

Liraz Shveka: *Souvenirs De La Nouvelle New Orleans*, Sidney Bechet

Devon Cooke: *Sweet Home Chicago*, Bob Harrisson

Leonard Krause: *Feeling Good*, Michael Bublé
Jill Grant: *Tobacco Road*, Junior Wells
Tristan Brightman: *Come on in My Kitchen*, Porterdavis
Vincent Wong: *Satisfied Mind*, Ben Harper
Alberto Escalante: *Billie Jean*, The Civil Wars
Kevin Selfe: *Hard Time Killing Floor Blues*, Skip James (1931)
Velody: *Summertime*, Ray Brown Trio with Gene Harris
Jenny Hauser: *Cry to Me*, Solomon Burke
Dean Mueller: *Do I Move You*, Nina Simone
Dan Nash: *St. James Infirmary*, Louis Armstrong
Curtis Salgado: *Hoochie Coochie Man*, Muddy Waters

REFERENCES

BLUES MUSIC & DANCING

Davis, Francis. *The History of the Blue*s. Boston: Da Capo Press, 2008.

Handy, W. C. *Father of the Blues: An Autobiography.* Boston: Da Capo Press, 1969.

Murray, Albert. *Stomping the Blue*s. Boston: Da Capo Press, 1989.

Steinberg, Jesse R., and Abrol Fairweather, eds. *Blues Philosophy for Everyone.* Hoboken, NJ: Wiley-Blackwell, 2012.

Stearns, Marshall, and Jean Stearns. *Jazz Dance: The Story of American Vernacular Danc*e. Boston: Da Capo Press, 1994.

MIND/BODY/SPIRIT

Bowman, Katy. *Move Your DNA: Restore Your Health Through Natural Movement.* Carlsborg, WA: Propriometrics Press, 2014.

Hay, Louise. *Heal Your Body.* Carlsbad, CA: Hay House, 1976.

Van der Kolk, Bessel. *The Body Keeps the Score.* New York: Penguin Books, 2014.

FILMS

Alive Inside (2014 Documentary) www.aliveinside.us
Inside the Dance (2016 Documentary) www.insidethedance.com

www.ingramcontent.com/pod-product-compliance
Lightning Source LLC
Chambersburg PA
CBHW071220290326
41931CB00037B/1486